C000298777

OXFORD HANDBOOKS IN EI
Series Editors   R. N. Illingworth, C. F

OXFORD HANDBOOKS IN EMERGENCY MEDICINE

This series has already established itself as the essential reference series for staff in A & E departments.

Each book begins with an introduction to the topic, including epidemiology where appropriate. The clinical presentation and the immediate practical management of common conditions are described in detail, enabling the casualty officer or nurse to deal with the problem on the spot. Where appropriate a specific course of action is recommended for each situation and alternatives discussed. Information is clearly laid out and easy to find—important for situations where swift action may be vital.

Details on when, how, and to whom to refer patients are covered, as well as the information required at referral, and what this information is used for. The management of the patient after referral to a specialist is also outlined.

The text of each book is supplemented with checklists, key points, clear diagrams illustrating practical procedures, and recommendations for further reading.

The Oxford Handbooks in Emergency Medicine are an invaluable resource for every member of the A & E team, written and edited by clinicians at the sharp end.

Maxillofacial and Dental Emergencies

John E. Hawkesford
Consultant in Oral and Maxillofacial
Surgery and Clinical Director,
Newcastle General Hospital
Newcastle upon Tyne

and

James G. Banks
Consultant in Accident/Emergency Medicine,
Dryburn Hospital, Durham

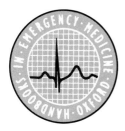

Oxford ● New York ● Tokyo
OXFORD UNIVERSITY PRESS
1994

Oxford University Press, Great Clarendon Street, Oxford OX2 6DP
Oxford New York
Athens Auckland Bangkok Bogota Bombay Buenos Aires
Calcutta Cape Town Dar es Salaam Delhi Florence Hong Kong Istanbul
Karachi Kuala Lumpur Madras Madrid Melbourne Mexico City
Nairobi Paris Singapore Taipei Tokyo Toronto Warsaw
and associated companies in
Berlin Ibadan

Oxford is a trade mark of Oxford University Press

Published in the United States
by Oxford University Press Inc., New York

© John E. Hawkesford and James G. Banks, 1994

First published in paperback 1994
Reprinted 1998

All rights reserved. No part of this publication may be
reproduced, stored in a retrieval system, or transmitted, in any
form or by any means, without the prior permission in writing of Oxford
University Press. Within the UK, exceptions are allowed in respect of any
fair dealing for the purpose of research or private study, or criticism or
review, as permitted under the Copyright, Designs and Patents Act, 1988, or
in the case of reprographic reproduction in accordance with the terms of
licences issued by the Copyright Licensing Agency. Enquiries concerning
reproduction outside those terms and in other countries should be sent to
the Rights Department, Oxford University Press, at the address above.

This book is sold subject to the condition that it shall not,
by way of trade or otherwise, be lent, re-sold, hired out, or otherwise
circulated without the publisher's prior consent in any form of binding
or cover other than that in which it is published and without a similar
condition including this condition being imposed
on the subsequent purchaser.

A catalogue record for this book is available from the British Library

Library of Congress Cataloging in Publication Data
Hawkesford, John E.
Maxillofacial and dental emergencies / John E. Hawkesford and James
G. Banks.
(Oxford handbooks in emergency medicine ; 7)
Includes bibliographical references.
1. Facial bones–Fractures–Handbooks, manuals, etc.   2. Teeth-
Wounds and injuries–Handbooks, manuals, etc.   3. Face–Wounds and
injuries–Handbooks, manuals, etc.   4. Surgical emergencies–
Handbooks, manuals, etc.   5. Dental emergencies–Handbooks,
manuals, etc.   I. Banks, James G.   II. Title.   III. Series.
[DNLM: 1. Maxillofacial Injuries–diagnosis–handbooks.   2.
Maxillofacial Injuries–therapy–handbooks.   3. Facial Bones–injuries–
handbooks. 4. Tooth–Injuries–handbooks.   5. Emergencies–
handbooks.   WB 39 098 v. 7 1993]
RD523.H39 1994   617.5'2044–dc20   93-24276
ISBN 0 19 261997 7 (Pbk)

Printed in Great Britain on acid-free paper by
Biddles Ltd, Guildford and King's Lynn

Preface

A significant number of patients with maxillofacial trauma or dental emergencies are seen in Accident and Emergency Departments. Many of these departments will not have an 'in-house' maxillofacial Surgery Department and Accident and Emergency staff will be required to assess the patient and provide initial treatment before referring the patient on to a specialist department. These patients will have various conditions, ranging from oral infections, dental trauma, and facial pain, to severe maxillofacial trauma and possible respiratory obstruction.

Most Accident and Emergency staff will have had very little training in diagnosis and treatment of dental and maxillofacial emergencies and the purpose of this handbook is to give them some understanding of and advice on the assessment and initial treatment of patients with such injuries.

Prompt diagnosis of these emergency patients, followed by appropriate management decisions, initial treatment, and prompt referral to the specialist Oral and Maxillofacial Surgery Department, will significantly affect the prognosis and reduce patient morbidity.

March 1994   J.E.H.
Newcastle upon Tyne   J.G.B.

Acknowledgements

We would like to thank the many past and present members of the Catherine Cookson Oral and Maxillofacial Surgery Department at Newcastle General Hospital who have helped in the preparation of this handbook and in particular to Dr Richard Welbury, Consultant in Paediatric Dentistry, for contributing to the chapter on dental pain, infection, haemorrhage, and trauma. We are grateful to Ash Songra for his contribution to the chapter on the assessment and management of mandibular fractures and dislocations of the temporomandibular joint, Alistair Smyth for his contribution to the chapter on the assessment and treatment of fractures of the middle third of the facial skeleton, Velupillai Ilankovan for his contribution to the chapter on assessment of malar fractures and orbital complications of facial trauma and Martin Telfer for his contribution to the chapter on oral medicine and salivary gland disease.

We would also like to thank Peter Grencis and Ann Young of the Department of Medical Photography and Illustration and Miss Mary Brown of Dryburn Hospital, Durham. We would also like to thank Robin Illingworth of St James University Hospital in Leeds and the staff at Oxford University Press for all their help and advice given.

Last but not least our thanks go to Miss Gillian Hopper of Newcastle General Hospital for typing the manuscript on many occasions.

Contents

Dose schedules are being continually revised and new side effects recognized. Oxford University Press makes no representation, express or implied, that the drug dosages in this book are correct. For these reasons the reader is strongly urged to consult the drug company's printed instructions before administering any of the drugs recommended in this book.

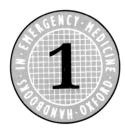

CHAPTER 1

Introduction

Epidemiology

- **Assaults   Road-traffic accidents   Sports injuries
  Dog bites   Other causes of facial injury**

Many patients attending accident and emergency departments have oral and maxillofacial injuries, accounting for 6 per cent of all new attenders in one study (Wood and Herion 1991).

In a review of the aetiology of maxillofacial fractures in the United Kingdom, Telfer *et al.* (1991) reported that in the decade 1977–87 there was a 20 per cent increase in the number of patients treated, and that, while there were fewer severe injuries, the number of patients injured in assaults had increased by 47 per cent, whilst the number injured in road-traffic accidents had decreased by 34 per cent.

Assaults

Facial injuries from assaults are typically seen in young men, especially at weekends. These patients are often drunk and uncooperative, making accurate clinical diagnosis difficult. Achieving a reduction of high alcohol intake, with its consequent aggressive behaviour, is a problem that the medical profession and society at large must tackle if the number of injuries from assaults is to fall.

Road-traffic accidents

The introduction of seat-belt legislation has been beneficial in reducing maxillofacial injuries in front-seat occupants. However, despite this welcome trend, Bradford *et al.* (1986) encountered a 28 per cent incidence of soft-tissue facial injuries and a 6 per cent incidence of facial fractures in occupants of vehicles involved in major road-traffic accidents. Soft-tissue injuries are principally caused by flying glass or direct contact with the windscreen or side window. The chances of being struck by flying glass are reduced if the windscreen is made of laminated rather than toughened glass. Facial contact with the steering wheel is also an important cause of soft-tissue injuries and, in addition, is the principle cause of fractures of the facial skeleton, principally involving the nasal bones, mandible, and zygoma.

These injuries to drivers would be reduced by the use of air bags, which inflate from the steering mechanism following impact, thus cushioning a blow to the driver's face. In the United Kingdom at the present time, air bags are increasingly being fitted in vehicles.

Sports injuries

Injuries to the head, face, and neck account for approximately 18 per cent of sports-related injuries (McLatchie 1986). Facial injuries may occur in sports such as boxing, rugby, ice hockey, and cricket. The incidence of such injuries is reduced by the use of appropriate faceguards, which are mandatory for fencers and goalkeepers in ice hockey, but still optional for cricketers. The wearing of a gum-shield is mandatory for boxers, and is also recommended in contact sports such as rugby and ice hockey. Almost 50 per cent of all eye injuries associated with sport are due to contact with a ball. The squash ball has received much attention in producing blow-out fractures of the orbit, and players are advised to wear safety goggles. Injuries to the pinna of the ear in rugby players may be reduced by the use of scrum caps or protective taping.

Dog bites

Although recent legislation has been introduced to control certain 'fighting dogs', bites can be sustained from dogs of any breed, and wounds to the face are particularly prevalent in children, often as the result of entering a dog's 'territory'. Other factors which are thought to increase the risk of being bitten by a dog include disturbing the animal while it is resting or sleeping, and excessive teasing or playing, which may lead to the dog becoming over-excited; dogs are more likely to bite than bitches. Young children as soon as they are old enough to understand should be taught to approach strange dogs with caution.

Other causes of facial injury

Falls on to the face are particularly prevalent amongst the elderly and the very young. Falls in the elderly may be reduced in some instances by appropriate treatment of any relevant underlying medical condition. Facial injury to young children can be reduced by encouraging their use of soft play-areas.

Clinical considerations

Facial trauma and dental emergencies often receive relatively little attention in the undergraduate medical curriculum. Junior casualty officers must be taught a clinical evaluation of the injured face, so that appropriate management decisions can be made. It is vitally important that adequate notes should be recorded, preferably with the use of diagrams or drawings, for example to demonstrate the anatomical site and length of wounds. This is not only important in a clinical context, but also for medico-legal reasons, particularly in cases of assault, where the examining doctor may be required to appear in court as a witness. Good clinical records are also needed for reports for insurance companies, for the Criminal Injuries Compensation Board, and for police statements. Also in a medico-legal context, facial injuries may preclude the use of the breathalyser in measuring alcohol levels. Under these circumstances, the police may request the presence of a police surgeon to obtain blood samples for alcohol measurement. If the police ask to use a breathalyser, the accident and emergency doctor should record whether or not the patient is fit to use it and understands the request.

Inappropriate management of dental trauma may have long-term consequences for the patient. Although most dentists now provide an out-of-hours emergency service, medical staff in accident and emergency departments must be aware of conditions which require urgent attention, with referral to the oral surgeon if appropriate, and others for which treatment can be started by the accident and emergency doctor, with subsequent referral on a less urgent basis.

The succeeding chapters in this book are concerned with the initial diagnosis and treatment of patients with maxillofacial and dental trauma, and give guidance as to when the maxillofacial specialist should be involved in further management.

Further reading

Bradford, M., Otubushin, A., Thomas, P., Robertson, N., and Green, P. D. (1986). Head and face injuries to car occupants in accidents/ field data 1983–1985. Presented at the International Conference on the Biomechanics of Impacts.

McLatchie, G. R. (1986). *Essentials of sports medicine*. Churchill Livingstone, Edinburgh.

Shewell, P. C. and Nancarrow, J. D. (1991). Dogs that bite. *British Medical Journal*, **303**, 1512–13.

Telfer, M. R., Jones, G. M., and Shepherd, J. P. (1991). Trends in the aetiology of maxillo-facial fractures in the United Kingdom (1977–1987). *British Journal of Oral and Maxillo-Facial Surgery*, **29**, 250–5.

Wood, G. D. and Herion, S. (1991). Oral and maxillo-facial surgery: should a district service be retained? *Archives of Emergency Medicine*, **8**, 257–62.

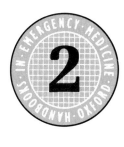

CHAPTER 2

Dental pain, infection, haemorrhage, and trauma

Richard Welbury

Key points in dental pain, infection, haemorrhage, and trauma

1 General Dental Practitioners throughout the UK run a 24-hours emergency service. This should be utilized for pain patients.

2 Dental infection if left untreated or treated too late and inadequately can be life-threatening.

3 Dental haemorrhage must be treated promptly. Early specialist referral should be sought if treatment in A & E is not successful.

4 Chest X-rays should be taken in all patients with missing teeth who have had a period of unconsciousness.

5 Displaced permanent teeth should be referred for immediate dental attention.

6 Avulsed permanent teeth brought in for implantation should be put back into their sockets and referred for immediate dental attention. Early reimplantation improves prognosis.

Applied anatomy: the oral cavity

- **Lips Cheeks Floor of the mouth Tongue Alveolar ridges and gingiva Palate**

The oral cavity extends from the lips to the palatoglossal fold. The roof is formed by the hard and soft palate, the lateral walls by the cheeks; the tongue projects upwards from the floor. Within these boundaries lie the upper and lower alveolar ridges and teeth. Keratinized mucous membrane (stratified squamous epithelium) lines the gingivae and hard palate, and non-keratinized mucous membrane the other areas, including the inner aspects of the lips and the floor of the mouth.

Lips

The bulk of the lips is made up of the orbicularis oris muscle, supplied by the VII (facial) cranial nerve. Other muscles of facial expression are inserted into parts of the orbicularis oris muscle.

The blood-supply to the upper lip is from the superior labial arteries, and that to the lower lip from the inferior labial arteries, both being branches of the facial arteries from the external carotids. Anastomoses occur across the midline. Drainage of blood is via the superior and inferior labial veins to the facial veins.

Cheeks

The bulk of the cheeks is made up of the buccinator muscle, which is attached behind to the outer aspect of the upper alveolus in the region of the molar teeth, to the external oblique line of the mandible, and to the pterygomandibular raphe between these two. It is inserted anteriorly into the lateral part of the orbicularis oris, and, like that muscle, is supplied by the facial nerve. The lining of the cheeks is of non-keratinized mucous membrane, apart from an area of keratinization which corresponds to the occlusal surfaces of the teeth.

The cheeks also contain a large quantity of fat tissue, and

have numerous salivary glands situated between the buccinator and the oral mucous membrane.

Floor of the mouth

This area is largely covered by the tongue, and is bounded
laterally and anteriorly by the teeth (Fig. 2.1).
The floor of the mouth is made up of the following paired
structures.

(1) the mylohyoid muscles;

(2) the genioglossus muscles;

(3) the geniohyoid muscles;

(4) the anterior bellies of the digastric muscles;

(5) the sublingual salivary glands and ducts;

(6) the submandibular salivary glands and ducts; and

(7) blood-vessels, nerves,and lymphatics.

    1. The mylohyoid muscles originate from the mylohyoid
line of the mandible, and their anterior fibres are inserted
into the body of the hyoid bone. The posterior fibres anasto-
mose with the muscle of the opposite side in the median
line. The submandibular salivary gland folds around the

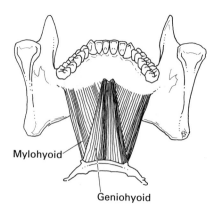

Fig. 2.1 • The main muscles of the floor of the mouth.

posterior free edge of the muscle, and this divides the gland into superficial (above the mylohyoid) and deep (below it) parts.

2. The genioglossus, a triangular-shaped muscle, originates from the superior genial tubercle of the mandible and spreads out to be inserted into the base of the tongue.

3. The geniohyoid, a narrow muscle, originates from the inferior genial tubercle and runs downwards and backwards to be inserted into the hyoid bone.

4. The digastric muscle has an anterior and a posterior belly. The anterior belly originates from the digastric fossa of the inferior border of the mandible. It is attached to the hyoid bone by a fibrous sling, and then continues backward as the posterior belly, which is inserted into the digastric notch in the mastoid process of the temporal bone.

Landmarks in the floor of the mouth on raising the tip of the tongue to touch the upper teeth are (Fig. 2.2):

(a) the lingual frenum, which connects the undersurface of the tongue to the floor of the mouth;

(b) the sublingual papilla, found on each side of the frenum, which is the opening for the duct from the submandibular salivary gland; and

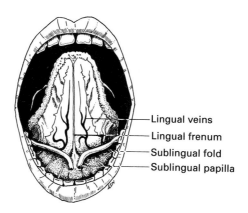

Fig. 2.2 • Landmarks of the floor of the mouth.

(c) the sublingual fold, which extends backwards and laterally in the floor of the mouth from the papilla, and has
minute openings in the surface from the ducts of the
sublingual salivary gland.

Tongue

The dorsum can be divided into the anterior two-thirds,
which lies in the oral cavity, and the posterior one-third,
which forms the anterior wall of the pharynx. Separating the
two parts is a shallow U-shaped furrow, the sulcus terminalis,
running outwards and forwards from a small midline pit, the
foramen caecum (Fig. 2.3).

The anterior two-thirds is covered with thick keratinized
epithelium; has three types of papillae on its surface,
filiform, fungiform, and vallate; and receives its sensory
supply from the lingual nerve, a branch of the mandibular
division of the trigeminal (Vth) cranial nerve.

The posterior one-third extends from the sulcus terminalis
to the epiglottis, is covered by thin non-keratinized epithelium with no papillae but a nodular appearance produced by
underlying lymphoid tissue, and receives its sensory supply
from the glossopharyngeal (IXth cranial) nerve.

Taste sensation from the anterior two-thirds travels initially
in the lingual nerve, but then passes via the chorda tympani

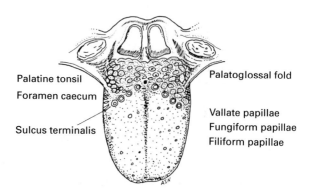

Fig. 2.3 • The dorsum of the tongue.

Palatine tonsil
Foramen caecum
Sulcus terminalis
Palatoglossal fold
Vallate papillae
Fungiform papillae
Filiform papillae

to the facial nerve. Taste from the posterior third travels in the glossopharyngeal nerve.

The muscles of the tongue are divided into two groups of four: the intrinsic muscles, which are contained entirely within the tongue, and the extrinsic muscles, which originate outside.

The intrinsic muscles are the superior and inferior longitudinal, vertical, and transverse muscles.

The extrinsic muscles of each side of the tongue are the genioglossus, hyoglossus, palatoglossus, and styloglossus.

1. The genioglossus—mentioned above. Its action is to pull the tongue forwards.

2. The hyoglossus arises from the hyoid bone and passes up to be inserted into the side of the tongue. It depresses the tongue.

3. The palatoglossus is a small, narrow muscle which arises from the aponeurosis of the soft palate and is inserted into the side of the tongue. It lifts up the tongue, closing off the mouth from the pharynx.

4. The styloglossus is a short muscle, originating on the styloid process and passing downwards and forwards to be inserted into the side of the tongue. It draws the tongue upwards and backwards.

The motor nerve supply to all the muscles of the tongue except the palatoglossus is the hypoglossal (XII) cranial nerve; the palatoglossus is supplied by the accessory (XI) cranial nerve.

The blood supply reaches the tongue via the lingual artery, a branch of the external carotid, and drains principally through the lingual vein.

Alveolar ridges and gingiva

The upper and lower alveolar ridges are covered by firmly adherent keratinized epithelium termed the gingiva. When healthy the gingiva is pale pink in colour, and may have diffuse areas of darker pigmentation in coloured races. Its surface is stippled, resembling the texture of orange peel.

The gingiva on the buccal aspect of the upper and lower

alveolus and the lingual aspect of the lower alveolus is continuous with the redder non-keratinized oral mucous membrane, and the clear line of demarcation between the two is called the mucogingival junction. The palatal gingiva of the upper alveolus merges imperceptibly with the pink keratinized epithelium covering the whole of the hard palate.

The gingivae are scalloped around the teeth, meeting between the teeth in a point, the interdental papilla. In a collar around the teeth is a narrow band of unstippled gingiva, the 'free' gingiva, which is not tightly bound down to the alveolar bone. This is demarcated from the attached gingiva by a shallow free gingival groove, which follows the outline of the gingival margin (Fig. 2.4).

Palate

The hard palate is formed by parts of the maxillae and palatine bones. It is lined by thick keratinized epithelium that is tightly bound down to underlying bone. The incisive papilla lies immediately behind the anterior teeth, and the median raphe, a hard ridge, runs posteriorly in the midline. In the anterior part of the palate a series of corrugations of the mucosa, the rugae, lie parallel to the anterior teeth.

The blood-supply to the hard palate is from the greater palatine artery through the greater palatine foramen. The nerve-supply is by two branches of the trigeminal (Vth) cranial nerve. The area immediately behind the anterior teeth is supplied by the nasopalatine nerve, but the greater part of the area is supplied by the anterior palatine nerve, which emerges via the greater palatine foramen.

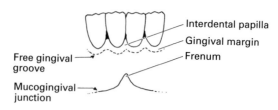

Fig. 2.4 • Landmarks around the teeth.

The soft palate extends backwards and downwards from the hard palate, and is mobile, functioning during swallowing to close off the nasopharynx from the oropharynx or during respiration to close off the oral cavity from the oropharynx.

Applied anatomy: the dentition

- **Terminology   General tooth structure   Chronology of eruption of teeth**

Human beings develop two complete sets of teeth in their lifetime: the primary (deciduous) dentition, commonly called the 'baby teeth' or 'milk teeth', and the permanent dentition, which replaces the primary one during childhood between 6 and 12 years of age. There are 20 primary and 32 permanent teeth.

Terminology

For identification purposes, the two dental arches are each divided into right and left halves, making four quadrants: upper right and left, and lower right and left. The five primary teeth in each quadrant are given the letters a to e, working backwards from the midline, and the eight permanent teeth of each quadrant are numbered 1 to 8 in a similar way (Figs 2.5 and 2.6).

Diagrammatically, the teeth are shown as follows:

$$\text{Primary dentition} = \frac{\text{e d c b a} \mid \text{a b c d e}}{\text{e d c b a} \mid \text{a b c d e}}$$

$$\text{Permanent dentition} = \frac{\text{8 7 6 5 4 3 2 1} \mid \text{1 2 3 4 5 6 7 8}}{\text{8 7 6 5 4 3 2 1} \mid \text{1 2 3 4 5 6 7 8}}$$

An upper left deciduous central will be designated $\mid \underline{a}$, a lower right permanent lateral incisor $\overline{2} \mid$, a lower left permanent third molar $\mid \overline{8}$, etc.

General tooth structure

Each tooth is composed of a crown and one or more roots.

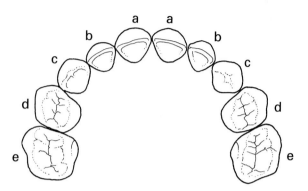

Fig. 2.5 • The primary upper arch.

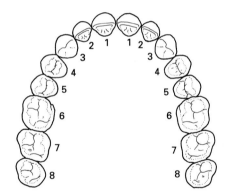

Fig. 2.6 • The permanent upper arch.

The bulk of the tooth is made up of dentine, but the crown is covered by a layer of enamel and the roots by a thin layer of cementum. The tooth has a hollow centre which contains the pulp (nerves and blood-vessels) (Figs. 2.7 and 2.8).

Primary teeth are smaller, whiter, and more bulbous than permanent teeth.

In describing the various tooth surfaces, the following terms are used:

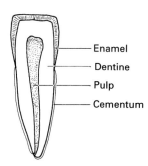

Fig. 2.7 • Structure of an incisor tooth.

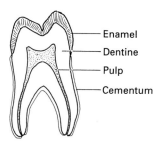

Fig. 2.8 • Structure of a molar tooth.

mesial	—	nearest the midline of the dental arch
distal	—	furthest from the midline
lingual	—	nearest the tongue
palatal	—	nearest the palate
labial	—	nearest the lips
buccal	—	nearest the cheeks
occlusal	—	the surface that comes into contact with the opposing teeth.

Chronology of eruption of teeth

There is a great deal of variation, and the eruption chronology given in Table 2.1 is based on normal averages.

Table 2.1 • Chronology of eruption of teeth

Tooth	Symbol	Eruption
Primary		
central	a	6 months
lateral	b	9 months
canine	c	18 months
first molar	d	12 months
second molar	e	24 months
Permanent		
central	1	6–7 years
lateral	2	8 years
canine	3	11 years
first premolar	4	9 years
second premolar	5	10 years
first molar	6	6 years
second molar	7	12 years
third molar	8	18–20 years

Primary
Calcification begins at approximately 6 months of fetal life. The roots are complete by 1–1½ years after eruption. Teeth are exfoliated or lost from the mouth about 6 months before their permanent successors are due to erupt.

Permanent
Calcification begins approximately 6 years before eruption (except canines, which begin 4 months after birth). The roots are completed 3 years after eruption.

Dental caries and pain

• Lost fillings and pain

Dental caries, or tooth decay, affects the calcified portion of the tooth, and gradually destroys enamel and dentine until the nerve pulp is exposed. The degree of pain accompanying a carious lesion varies from extreme to none at all. Normally the degree of pain felt at each progression of caries is as follows (Fig. 2.9).

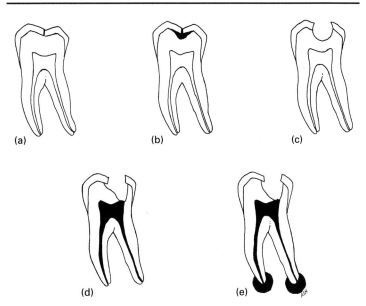

Fig. 2.9 • Diagram of the stages of carious breakdown of a lower molar tooth.

(a) The small pit where the enamel is still macroscopically intact is usually painless.

(b) A bluish-white coloured area where the enamel is still macroscopically intact will indicate a tooth that is sensitive to hot and cold stimulation.

(c) The open cavity with exposed dentine is generally painful on contact with hot, cold, and occasionally sweet foodstuffs. However, some quite large cavities are painless, either because the dentine is insulated by a layer of caries or food debris, or because the nerve has already died.

(d) Pulpitis presents as a severe throbbing pain, which is made worse by heat, and tends to be eased by cold. When the inflammation associated with caries reaches the pulp it cannot swell because of its enclosure within hard calcified dentine, so the pressure builds up, causing a throbbing pain.

(e) An acute apical abscess causes a throbbing pain due to pressure building up in the periapical tissues. It is increased by pressing the tooth into the socket (for example by biting or tapping). Eventually the pus discharges, either through the open pulp into the mouth (if the tooth is grossly decayed) or through the alveolar bone. In either case, as long as discharge can occur, the abscess becomes chronic and relatively painless. In many cases, therefore, the acute and painful phase does not occur.

Pain originating from dental caries requires the attention of a Dental Surgeon to eradicate the cause and to either restore, restore and root-fill, or extract the tooth. All areas of the United Kingdom should now have Dental Practitioners advertising evening and 24-hour emergency services in the Yellow Pages. This should be drawn to the attention of the patient attending A & E, and this avenue of help should be explored. However, when professional dental help is not forthcoming the patient with a pulpitis or an apical abscess should be prescribed an antibiotic (penicillin 250–500 mg four times a day) and an analgesic (aspirin 300–900 mg four times a day, or an NSAI, for instance ibuprofen 400 mg four times a day) and advised to see a dentist as soon as possible. Erythromycin is an alternative antibiotic in patients allergic to penicillin. Tetracycline should never be prescribed to anyone under 10 years of age, because of the risk of intrinsic staining in developing teeth. Aspirin has been shown to be the most affective analgesia for dental pain, but should be used with the usual precautions. Contrary to popular belief, opioid analgesics are not very effective in the relief of dental pain.

Lost fillings and pain

When a filling or part of a filling has been lost pain may be due to thermal stimulation of exposed dentine, or to caries, or to both. If a dentist is not available and there is a dental emergency box in the A & E department the defect can be filled with a temporary filling material based on zinc oxide and eugenol. One type of temporary material is dispensed ready mixed in a tube (Cavit-E), and, after drying the tooth as well as possible, this can pressed into position with a dental 'flat plastic' instrument (Fig. 2.10a). Other temporary filling materials, however, will need to be mixed by hand from powder and liquid dispenser bottles (for example, Kalzinol or Sedanol). The recommended powder: liquid ratio for these is of the order 5:1 by weight. On to a clean glass slab tap out 1 cm^2 of powder from its bottle, and then two drops of liquid from its dispenser bottle (keep them apart). Incorporate successive small portions of powder into the liquid with a spatula (Fig. 2.10b), ensuring complete mixing after each addition. Continue adding powder until a putty-like consistency is obtained. Mixing time should be about 1–1½ minutes, and the working time is 2 minutes from the end of

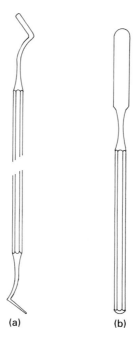

(a) (b)

Fig. 2.10 • (a) The 'flat plastic' dental instrument; (b) spatula for mixing dental cement.

the mix. To prevent the cement sticking to the instrument during placement dip the tip into the surplus powder on the mixing slab. The cement will set approximately 3 minutes after insertion in the mouth, and any excess can be gently removed with the 'flat plastic' instrument.

If these teeth are not sensitive to percussion (tapping on the tooth) and there are no signs of apical infection then an antibiotic should not be prescribed, and the patient should be instructed to see a dentist as soon as possible and to avoid eating or drinking anything very hot or very cold.

Orofacial infections

- **Symptoms and signs   Treatment   Osteomyelitis Dry socket**

Dental disease is the underlying cause of most of the inflammatory swellings which occur either in or around the jaws.

Inflammation may commence at the root apices or gingival margins of erupted teeth, in the soft tissues that surround and overlie the crowns of unerupted or partially erupted teeth, or, more rarely, in the jaw bones themselves (osteomyelitis). Inflammation around the apices of the tooth roots usually results in the formation of pus. This will take the line of least resistance, before perforating bone at its weakest and thinnest point, to involve the surrounding soft tissue, where it may either resolve, become localized, or spread. Spreading infections can both spread along and be limited by muscle and fascial planes.

The points of bony weakness vary in differing areas of the jaws, and some of the directions in which pus, formed in a periapical lesion, may spread into the surrounding soft tissues are illustrated in Fig. 2.11.

If pus perforates either the maxillary or the mandibular buccal plate it presents intraorally if it is inside the bony attachment of the buccinator muscle, and extraorally if outside it. When mandibular pus perforates lingually it presents intraorally if the apices of the teeth lie above the bony attach-

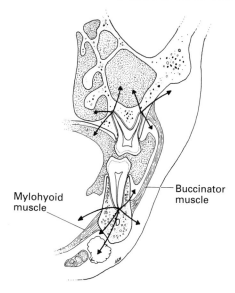

Fig. 2.11 • Direction in which pus formed in a periapical lesion may track.

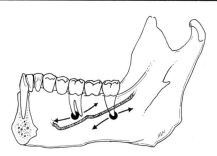

Fig. 2.12 • The lingual spread of pus from apical infections on lower molars, showing the relationship of the teeth to the mylohyoid muscle.

ment of the mylohyoid muscle (incisors, canines, and pre-molars), and extraorally if they lie below it (second and third molars) (Fig. 2.12). Apical infection from the first molar tooth is notoriously variable in its presentation.

The head and neck region has a number of fascial planes, and therefore a number of potential fascial spaces. These spaces intercommunicate, and although infection when present is rarely limited to one space it is important to know the boundaries and contents of these potential spaces.

Superficial sublingual space: between the oral mucosa of the floor of the mouth and the underlying mylohyoid muscle.

Deep sublingual space: between the mylohyoid muscle and the layer of deep cervical fascia which separates that muscle from the submandibular salivary gland.

Submandibular space: contains the submandibular salivary gland and is enclosed by the two layers of deep fascia, which are derived from the investing layer of the cervical fascia below and are attached above to the inner surface and the lower border of the mandible.

The sublingual spaces communicate with each other and with the submandibular space, and the submandibular space communicates with the pharyngeal spaces.

When infection spreads posteriorly from the mandibular molar region (Fig. 2.13) it can pass either buccally or lingually to the ascending ramus. If it passes buccally it can either spread between the masseter muscle and the skin and superficial fascia overlying it, or extend subperiosteally beneath the masseteric attachment into the *submasseteric space*. If infection passes lingually it reaches the *lateral pharyngeal space*, which is bounded anteriorly by the pterygomandibular raphe, posteriorly by the styloid process and its attached muscles, laterally by the medial pterygoid muscle, the ascending ramus of the mandible, and the deep surface of the parotid gland, and medially by the cervical fascia covering the outer surface of the superior constrictor muscle. Infection in the lateral pharyngeal space may spread upwards to the base of the skull, downwards to the glottis, or into the mediastinum. The dangerous complications of cavernous sinus thrombosis, glottic oedema, or mediastinitis illustrate the importance of prompt treatment of infection in this space. Infection may originate from mandibular molars,

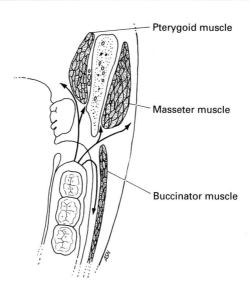

Fig. 2.13 • Directions in which pus may track backwards from the mandibular molar region.

the submandibular space, or, rarely, medial rupture of an infected parotid gland.

Periapical infections arising in maxillary incisor and canine teeth may spread into the upper lip and canine fossa. If the infection gains entry into the superior labial venous plexus it may spread via the facial and angular veins and enter the cranium, causing cavernous sinus thrombosis. Similarly, acute soft-tissue infections of the infra-orbital region of the cheek may rapidly become dangerous unless effective treatment is instituted promptly.

Symptoms and signs of orofacial infections

The patient may complain of pain, feeling hot, general malaise, inability to open the mouth fully (trismus), difficulty in swallowing (dysphagia) and pain on swallowing, difficulty in speaking, and in extreme cases difficulty in breathing. Signs of infection may range from localized swellings in the buccal sulcus or palate adjacent to a tooth, to the frank facial asymmetry of submandibular cellulitis, with a tense warm swelling extraorally and an elevated floor of mouth and dorsum of tongue intraorally.

Treatment of orofacial infections

Patients with localized swellings related to one tooth with a recent history of pain in that tooth who have little or no trismus or systemic signs of infection should be referred directly to a general dental practitioner. If one is not available then the patient should be placed on penicillin (erythromycin if allergic) 250/500 mg four times a day and instructed to attend a dentist the next day or after the weekend.

Patients with either significant trismus, dysphagia, respiratory distress, or systemic toxicity should be referred immediately to the nearest oral and maxillofacial surgery department for admission, where treatment will include systemic antibiotics (versus aerobes and anaerobes) and surgery.

Patients with suspected cavernous sinus thrombosis, require immediate referral to a neurosurgical unit.

Osteomyelitis

This condition is not as prevalent as it was, which is probably attributable to improved dental hygiene. The mandible is more commonly affected, owing to its poorer vascularity.

The condition is characterized by marked pyrexia and pain and by tenderness to extra-oral palpation. The onset of impairment of labial sensation some hours or days after extraction of a tooth is synonymous with acute osteomyelitis. These patients require emergency admission to an oral and maxillofacial surgery department.

Dry socket

This is a well-recognized complication of tooth extraction, but its aetiology is still not clear. It is usually regarded as a localized osteitis involving the lamina dura lining a tooth socket. The condition is characterized by an acutely painful tooth socket containing bare bone and broken-down blood-clot. Mandibular extractions are complicated by the development of a dry socket more frequently than maxillary extractions, and this may also be due to the greater density and poorer vascularity of the mandible.

Treatment by the dentist involves local socket irrigation plus debridement, bone-trimming, and placement of a loose zinc–oil of cloves dressing into the socket. Should a dentist not be available the casualty officer should prescribe analgesia (aspirin or an NSAI) and warm saline mouthwashes (1 tsp salt in 30 ml water four times a day). True dry socket does not usually require antibiotics; but in the absence of dental help the casualty officer should prescribe penicillin (erythromycin) 250 mg four times a day.

Haemorrhage after tooth extraction

- **Management**

A common dental emergency is bleeding following the extraction of a tooth. The bleeding occurs usually from the alveolar mucosa around the rim of the tooth socket rather than from the socket itself.

Management of dental haemorrhage

1. Remove the excess blood-clot from the bleeding area with a piece of gauze.

2. Roll up a piece of gauze into a fat cigar shape, place it over the socket, and instruct the patient to bite on it. Leave for 10 minutes before checking.

3. If this is unsuccessful, or if there is a tear in the gum margins, a horizontal mattress suture under local analgesia will be required (Fig. 2.14a,b). In dentistry local analgesia is usually obtained using 2 per cent lignocaine with 1:80 000 adrenaline vasoconstrictor. The adrenaline reduces bleeding into the operating field. However, if only 2 per cent lignocaine is available this will suffice. In the upper arch 1 ml of local anaesthetic solution should be deposited buccally adjacent to the bleeding socket by inserting the needle just beneath the mucous membrane

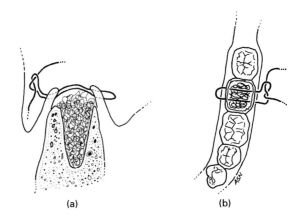

Fig. 2.14 • Horizontal mattress suture used for bleeding sockets (a and b).

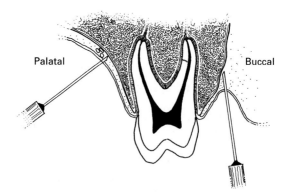

Fig. 2.15 • Buccal and palatal infiltrations in the upper arch.

where the mucosa reflects to line the cheeks, and 0.5 ml of solution submucosally palatal to the socket about 1 cm from the gum margin (Fig. 2.15). In the lower arch 1 ml of local anaesthetic solution should be deposited buccal to the bleeding socket at the mucosal reflection, and a further 1 ml lingually into the floor of the mouth between the alveolar mucosal reflection and the sublingual papilla. The object of the horizontal mattress suture is not to close the socket by approximating the soft tissues over it, but to tense the mucoperiosteum over the underlying bone so that it becomes ischaemic. The suture materials most commonly used are 3/0 silk, 3/0 vicryl or 3/0 softgut. Vicryl and softgut are resorbable, the latter rather more quickly than the former. After suturing get the patient to bite on rolled gauze again for 10 minutes.

4. Should these measures fail to control haemorrhage then pack 1 cm^2 of oxidized cellulose gauze (Surgicel) into the wound under the mattress suture. The patient should bite for a further 10 minutes on rolled gauze. If this fails to control haemorrhage the patient should be referred to the nearest oral surgery department for further treatment.

After the haemorrhage has stopped the patient should be instructed not to take repeated or vigorous rinses, and to avoid eating food likely to disturb the clot, for example crisps or peanuts, and to attend his or her dentist for a check-up the following day.

Fractured and missing teeth

If all or part of a tooth is missing in a patient who has been unconscious then a chest X-ray must be taken in case it has been inhaled into the lungs.

Fractures of anterior teeth are common, especially as a result of falls during play, fights, and contact sports. These injuries can be painful if a large area of dentine is exposed, and especially if the nerve of the tooth is exposed: this is readily seen as a red spot in the centre of the fracture line (Fig. 2.16c). Such injuries should be referred to a dentist, who will extirpate the pulp (remove the nerve remnants) under local anaesthetic to give immediate relief of pain. If dental help is not available the tooth may be dressed with zinc oxide-eugenol temporary cement after buccal infiltration of 2 ml of local anaesthetic solution. However, because the cement is not adhesive to the tooth substance it will need

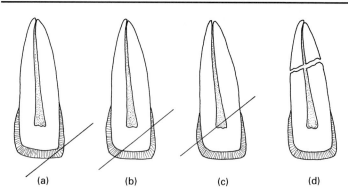

Fig. 2.16 • Simple classification for tooth fractures.
(a) Enamel only; (b) Enamel and dentine; (c) Enamel, dentine, and pulp;
(d) Root fracture.

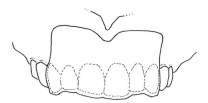

Fig. 2.17 • Soft metal-cement temporary splint.

to be protected by a splint. A convenient source of soft metal available is a milk-bottle top, and this can be fashioned as follows (Fig. 2.17):

1. Cut the metal to size, long enough to extend over two or three teeth on either side of the fractured tooth and wide enough to extend over the incisal edges and 3–4 mm over the labial and palatal gingiva.

2. Place the metal over the teeth and bend it down over the labial and palatal surfaces. Note where it is unnecessarily over-extended, remove it from the mouth, and modify its shape accordingly.

3. Replace the metal over the teeth and, with gentle finger pressure, adapt it as closely as possible to the teeth labially and palatally.
4. Cement the metal to the teeth with a more runny mix of zinc oxide–eugenol cement than that described in the 'lost fillings' section.

Subluxed (displaced) teeth

Subluxed teeth are ones that are displaced from their normal position but still retained in their sockets.

Primary teeth are usually very mobile when subluxed, and this will not improve even if they are repositioned. The potential danger to the airway of the young child far outweighs any aesthetic considerations, and it is advisable that displaced mobile primary teeth are extracted.

On the other hand every attempt should be made to retain displaced permanent anterior teeth. The prognosis for these teeth depends on the severity of the primary injury and also on the speed at which dental help is obtained. If an oral surgeon or dentist is not available quickly then A & E staff should attempt repositioning and splinting.

1. Infiltrate buccally and palatally (lingually) as previously described.
2. Hold the displaced tooth between thumb and forefinger, and press gently back into the correct position; then compress the socket around the tooth for 1 minute.
3. Either fashion a 'milk-bottle top' splint and cement in place as previously described (Fig. 2.17), or if available use an adhesive bandage temporary splint. A proprietary material is available (Stomahesive, Squibb), composed of pectin, gelatin, carboxymethylcellulose, and polyisobutylene, which is sandwiched between a smooth polyethylene film on one side and a removable backing paper on the other. It adheres to moist hard or soft tissues, and gradually disintegrates in the mouth; within 24 to 72 hours it completely disappears or is reduced to small remnants which are easily removed.

(a) Before removing the backing paper, cut a piece similar in shape to that described for the soft metal splint.

(b) Adapt one half of the bandage to the labial surfaces (Fig. 2.18a), and then bend it over the incisal edges of the teeth on to the palatal surfaces (Fig. 2.18b). Modify its shape as necessary.

(c) Remove the backing paper and place the bandage on the moist teeth and gingiva; the material is hydrophilic and therefore adheres to moist surfaces. Use finger pressure to adapt it as closely as possible, and then use a flat plastic instrument to push it interdentally.

4. If the patient cannot be seen by a dentist for a few hours commence oral penicillin (erythromycin) 250 mg four times a day.

Reimplantation of avulsed teeth

• **Telephone advice   Immediate treatment in hospital**

Reimplantation of anterior primary teeth is not indicated because of extreme mobility and splinting problems; but

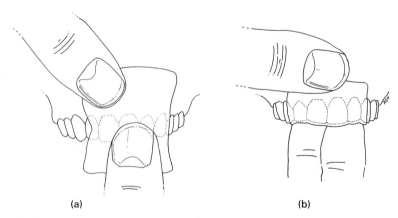

(a)   (b)

Fig. 2.18 • Adhesive bandage temporary splint (a and b).

reimplantation of anterior permanent teeth is simple, and has a good success rate if done promptly and correctly.

1. *Telephone advice*

   Tell the patient to clean the tooth by sucking it or by washing in milk and replant immediately into its socket, keeping it in place by finger pressure or by lightly biting on a handkerchief, and to attend a dental practice or a hospital as soon as possible. If this is not possible the best storage medium is saliva, placing the tooth in the buccal sulcus against the cheek; alternatively put it in a glass of milk. Avoid tap-water or disinfectant. If the patient has suffered a head injury as a result of the accident the tooth should not be replanted or carried in the buccal sulcus. The risk of again dislodging and inhaling a replanted tooth in someone with an impaired conscious level is high.

2. *Immediate treatment in hospital*

   A history of rheumatic fever, septal defects, valvular heart disease, previous valvular surgery, and immuno-suppressive drug therapy are all contraindications to reimplantation. The potential morbidity and mortality from subacute bacterial endocarditis far outweighs the aesthetic disadvantage of losing an anterior tooth. If in doubt discuss with an oral surgeon.

   (a) Hold the tooth by its crown and gently remove any dirt with gauze soaked in normal saline. Check for root fractures; if present, do not reimplant.

   (b) Replace the tooth into its socket, gradually pushing it fully home. Prior evacuation of any blood clot in the socket and local analgesia are not usually required.

   (c) Compress the socket around the tooth between fore-finger and thumb for 1 minute.

   (d) If an oral surgeon or dentist is available the patient should be referred immediately, and kept biting gently on a rolled gauze swab until transfer.

   (e) If no dental help is at hand then either a 'milk-bottle top' or a stomahesive splint should be fitted, as previously described (Figs 2.17, 2.18).

(f) Tetanus prophylaxis status should be checked and prophylaxis given if necessary, together with oral penicillin (erythromycin) 250 ml four times a day.

(g) Dental referral should take place as soon as possible.

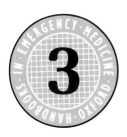

CHAPTER 3

Soft-tissue facial injuries

Key points in soft-tissue facial injuries

1 Most simple facial wounds can be closed in the accident and emergency department, although layered closure may be required, and suturing technique requires great care.
2 Consider the possibility of damage to deeper structures, for example the facial nerve or the parotid duct.
3 Wounds at certain sites require specialist referral—for example, the eyelid margin.
4 Ingrained abrasions must be properly cleaned and debrided.
5 Antibiotics are required for bites and contaminated wounds.

General introduction and indications for specialist referral

Facial appearance and expression form an important means of interpersonal communication. Soft-tissue injuries of the face cause concern and distress to patients and also to their relatives, who often worry about scarring or disfigurement. Injuries to the soft tissues of the face require meticulous repair to achieve the best functional and cosmetic results.

Wounds to the face are common in all age-groups, and the majority can be satisfactorily dealt with in the accident and emergency department, provided that sufficient care is taken. Wounds can range in severity from minor abrasions to major skin and muscle loss, with damage to underlying vessels, nerves, and salivary glands. These more extensive soft-tissue injuries are often associated with fractures of the facial skeleton, and require the special skills of the maxillofacial surgeon.

Box 3.1 Indications for primary referral to the maxillo-facial surgeon

- The wound is deep and may involve damage to the facial nerve, major vessels, or the parotid gland and/or duct.
- Wounds at special sites, for example involving the eyelid margins.
- There are deeply-embedded foreign bodies present.
- There is skin loss which may require the use of skin grafts or the mobilization of a local rotational skin flap.
- Specialist referral will lead to a significantly better cosmetic result than can be achieved in the accident and emergency department.

Clinical assessment

- History   Clinical and radiological examination

History

A clear history of how a facial wound has been sustained should be obtained from the patient, a parent, or a witness. This should alert the doctor to the likely extent of tissue damage and possible complications.

Box 3.2 **Important points in the history**

- Associated injuries to the head and cervical spine should be considered when the face has sustained a major impact, especially when there is associated loss of consciousness, and a patent airway should be ensured.
- The presence of foreign bodies should be suspected in certain circumstances, for example a shattered car windscreen.
- Damage to deep-lying structures should be suspected in cases of assault with a sharp instrument.
- Infection is a likely complication following bites or neglected wounds that are sometimes several hours or even days old.
- The possibility of non-accidental injury should be suspected in children with, for example, a torn labial frenulum, often associated with fingermark bruising on the skin.

Clinical and radiological examination

The correct approach to management is based on a thorough examination of the facial wound. The clinical findings should be clearly recorded.

X-ray examination should be performed *before* wound exploration and repair whenever the presence of foreign bodies or facial fracture is suspected on clinical grounds. Radio-

---

Box 3.3 **Important points in examination**

- The anatomical site. Consider damage to deep structures and ease of repair.
- The wound size (record in centimetres). The size of the wound may determine the best mode of repair and whether local or general anaesthetic is required.
- The wound depth should be assessed on initial examination, although it is often difficult to determine this accurately until local or general anaesthesia has been administered.
- Assess the degree of wound contamination. Wound debridement may be required.
- Assess possible damage to deep-lying structures, for instance bone, muscle, nerve, blood-vessel, parotid gland or duct, eyes, or lacrimal duct.

---

opaque foreign bodies in the soft tissues are poorly visualized on the standard facial views, and tangential views may be required. Patient co-operation is required to obtain films of diagnostic quality, and X-ray examination may have to be delayed until, for example, cerebral hypoxia has been corrected, or the effects of alcohol intoxication have diminished.

Management of facial wounds: anaesthesia

- **Surface anaesthesia   Local Anaesthesia
  Sedation   Local nerve blocks   General anaesthesia**

With the exception of very superficial wounds, adequate wound inspection, mechanical cleansing, and closure by sutures should be performed only after the administration of some form of anaesthetic. The choice of anaesthetic technique to be used should always be explained to the patient or to the parents of a child before the anaesthetic's administration.

Surface anaesthesia

Lignocaine gel will provide local anaesthesia on the skin surface. Its principal use in facial trauma is in the cleaning of superficial abrasions. After application it should be left for a period of 20 to 30 minutes in order to obtain maximum anaesthesia.

Local anaesthesia

The vast majority of facial wounds can be anaesthetized by injection of 1 per cent plain lignocaine around the wound, using a fine needle. The pain associated with puncture of the skin can be avoided if the needle is passed from within the wound subcutaneously until complete anaesthesia is achieved. The injection of lignocaine causes some initial pain, and the patient should be warned of this. Lignocaine with adrenaline is recommended if several wounds are to be closed under local anaesthetic. The adrenaline produces capillary constriction, delaying the absorption of the lignocaine and allowing larger doses to be used. An additional advantage is the reduction in capillary bleeding during wound cleansing.

Sedation

Although local anaesthetic infiltration is extremely effective, the injections required may be particularly distressing to young children, and may result in subsequent struggling, making the job of wound repair almost impossible. The administration of oral morphine in a dose of 0.1–0.2 mg/kg to an anxious child will have beneficial sedative and analgesic effect within about 30 minutes, thus enabling wound repair to be performed more easily. Intramuscular or intravenous midazolam 1.5–7.5 mg is a useful sedative in adults.

Local nerve blocks

Injection of lignocaine directly adjacent to the supraorbital, infraorbital, or mental nerves will produce anaesthesia of the forehead, cheek, and lower lip respectively. The technique requires a certain amount of practice and expertise. The techniques are well described in local anaesthetic textbooks.

General anaesthesia

Repair of facial wounds under general anaesthetic is indicated where the patient's co-operation cannot be guaranteed, for example, in distressed children and the mentally handicapped. General anaesthesia should be used when facial wounds are multiple and extensive, or there are injuries elsewhere which require surgical treatment.

Repair of facial wounds

- **Wound cleansing Foreign bodies Suturing technique Adhesive tapes Tetanus toxoid Antibiotics**

Wound cleansing

After suitable anaesthesia has been achieved, all wounds should be thoroughly cleaned with swabs soaked in saline or savlodil solution. Deeper wounds should be irrigated with a syringe containing normal saline solution. Gentle scrubbing of the wound may be required (a sterile toothbrush is useful for this procedure).

Foreign bodies

The wound should be thoroughly examined for the presence of foreign bodies, and any particulate matter should be lifted out with fine forceps. Glass foreign bodies, if previously visualized on X-ray, should be sought and removed from the wound before closure. Deeply-embedded foreign bodies which require further dissection for removal are better dealt with by the maxillofacial surgeon. If there is no on-site maxillofacial service and the patient has other more serious injuries requiring surgical attention, there may be no alternative but to close the facial wounds, leaving the foreign bodies to be removed electively at a later stage.

Suturing technique

The depth of the wound should be carefully assessed to determine whether the facial muscle has been divided. If this is the case, fine absorbable sutures should be used to repair the muscle. As the facial muscles of expression are closely related to the overlying skin, failure to repair any defect in the muscle layer may lead to the development of an unsightly sunken scar. While untidy skin edges can be trimmed with a scalpel or fine scissors, a general rule when dealing with facial wounds is to preserve as much skin as possible, as the vascularity of the facial tissues will normally ensure good healing.

When skin loss has occurred in association with a facial wound, mobilization of a local rotational skin flap or application of a full-thickness skin graft is often required. It is important to determine that there has been actual loss of skin, as this can be simulated by retraction of the wound edges. Repair of wounds with skin loss is the province of the plastic or maxillofacial surgeon, and should not be attempted in the accident and emergency department.

Adhesive tapes

Not all facial lacerations require suturing: some superficial wounds can be closed satisfactorily with adhesive tapes (for example Steristrips, 3M) with an acceptable cosmetic result. Adhesive tapes are particularly useful in superficial wounds of the forehead in children. They are, however, of little value in wounds near the eye, since they are often dislodged by movement. They should generally not be used on wounds of the chin, which are often much deeper than they initially appear. Histoacryl glue may often be used instead of adhesive tapes in wounds which are superficial and well away from the eyes.

After wound closure, most wounds can be left quite satisfactorily without any form of dressing. It should be remembered that elastoplast dressings are of little value on the 'beard area' in men. A dry dressing with an adhesive covering (for example Hypofix) is useful in children to prevent them handling the wound. Pressure dressings are

Box 3.4 **Points to remember when closing facial wounds**

- Fine instruments should be used for the closure of facial wounds, and, in particular, non-toothed forceps are preferable to toothed forceps, which may traumatize the tissues further.
- The use of fine, for example metric gauge 5/0 or 6/0 monofilament suture material, used with a small needle is preferable to the use of braided material, for example silk, as the former produces less tissue reaction.
- When closing an irregularly shaped wound, equivalent skin landmarks should be noted on either side of the wound. Insertion of the initial sutures through these points will prevent the skin distortion which may occur through suturing from one end of the wound to the other. Anatomical landmarks which may assist the surgeon are the vermilion in wounds of the lip, and the eyebrow, which should not be shaved, in wounds of the supra-orbital region.
- The sutures should always be passed from the free skin edge to the fixed one.
- The needle should always be inserted from the thinner tissue to the thicker, to ensure that the skin surface is level.
- Care should be taken to achieve the correct tension in the sutures to avoid skin overlap or inversion of the wound edges.
- Sutures should be removed within five days of wound repair. The early removal of sutures prevents 'pock mark' scars from the sutures. If there is concern that the wound may reopen after suture removal, adhesive tapes can be applied.

sometimes required after repair of wounds of the forehead with associated haematoma formation, once significant bleeding vessels have been ligated.

Tetanus toxoid

Enquiry should always be made regarding the patient's tetanus immune status. A tetanus toxoid booster should be administered to those who have not been vaccinated within ten years, with, for those with no history of immunization at any time the addition of an injection of human tetanus immunoglobulin (humotet) in cases where the wound has been sustained more than six hours before closure, or is contaminated.

Antibiotics

Antibiotics are not routinely required after wound closure, except in cases of bites (see below) or where the wound has been neglected and is frankly infected at the time of initial presentation. In the latter situation a swab should be taken, the wound should be irrigated, and a dressing should be applied. The most likely infective organism is *Staphylococcus aureus*, and a course of oral flucloxacillin should be started. The patient should be reviewed after 48 hours, and delayed primary closure should be considered at that time if the wound appears clean.

Special considerations

- **Skin abrasions Dog bites Airgun pellet wounds Wounds to the lip and contents of the oral cavity Wounds to the eyelid margins Injuries to the external ear Injury to the facial nerve Damage to sensory nerves Parotid gland and duct Facial infections**

Skin abrasions

Skin abrasions are usually the result of a fall on to the ground, often from pedal-cycles. The common mistake in

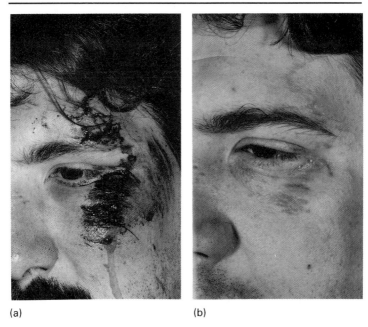

(a)   (b)

Fig. 3.1 • Ingrained abrasions of the left upper cheek, (a) before and (b) 3 months after initial treatment. Further surgery was required to excise the small areas of tattooed skin.

management of these injuries is failure to remove ingrained dirt, resulting in unsightly tattooing of the skin (Fig. 3.1). Small abrasions can usually be dealt with satisfactorily under local anaesthetic, but larger areas normally require a general anaesthetic. The abrasions should be thoroughly scrubbed to remove any loose particles, and a scalpel blade will be required to excise dirt-ingrained tissue. Provided adequate debridement is carried out, the final cosmetic result should be acceptable.

Dog bites

Dog bites to the face are normally seen in young children, and deserve special mention as the wounds are contaminated with bacteria from the animal's mouth. Unlike dog-bite wounds elsewhere on the body, those on the face should usually be closed by suturing after careful exploration and cleansing. A broad-spectrum antibiotic (for example augmentin) should be prescribed. Delayed primary closure of facial wounds is likely to result in less satisfactory scars than those achieved with immediate closure. Where dog bites have resulted in loss of tissue, referral of the patient to the plastic surgeon is appropriate.

Airgun pellet wounds

Penetrating injuries from airgun pellets are commonly seen in accident and emergency departments, and the face and head are often involved. The pellet may be felt subcutaneously several centimetres from the entry wound (Fig. 3.2). A pellet can be assumed to have penetrated deeply when it is not palpable and/or X-ray examination reveals deformity of the pellet, indicating contact with bone. Deeply-embedded pellets are best removed by the maxillofacial surgeon, but those lying more superficially can generally be removed in the accident and emergency department under local anaesthetic.

Wounds to the lip and contents of the oral cavity

Partial-thickness wounds to the external surface of the lip can be sutured in the usual manner under local anaesthetic. It is important that the first suture approximates the vermilion accurately, otherwise a cosmetically unacceptable step will be visible in the subsequent scar. Full-thickness wounds of the lip require closure in layers, absorbable sutures being used to close the mucosa and muscle layers, and a fine monofilament suture for the skin. Full-thickness wounds are better repaired by the maxillofacial or plastic surgeon. Small through-and-through wounds of upper and lower lip are normally caused by penetration from the incisor or canine teeth. If part of one of these teeth is missing, it may be embedded in the wound, and exploration will be required to remove it. Many of these wounds are very small, and do not require closure. Larger wounds should be closed with an absorbable suture to the mucosa and muscle

(a)

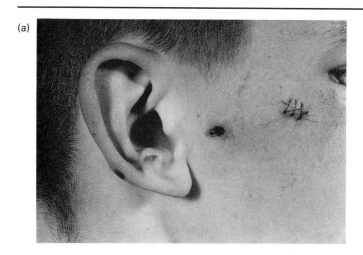

(b)

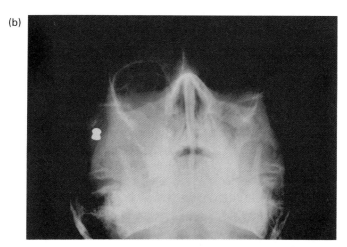

Fig. 3.2 • Airgun pellet injury, showing entry point on the posterior aspect of the pinna and further trajectory to final position overlying the zygoma. The upper illustration was taken after surgical removal of the pellet.

(for example 3/0 Vicryl) and a fine monofilament suture to the skin.

Degloving injuries of the labial mucosa from the base of the labial sulcus should be referred to the maxillofacial surgeon for repair.

Wounds of the tongue normally result from the forceful biting action of the teeth, for example after a fall on to the chin or a punch. Small transverse wounds of the tongue appear wide when the tongue is protruded, but the wound edges are closely apposed when the tongue is retracted. They will normally heal without the need for surgical repair. Wounds which are more extensive or involve the full thickness of the tongue should be referred to the maxillofacial surgeon for suturing.

Full-thickness wounds through the cheek to the buccal mucosa may result in profuse haemorrhage from branches of the facial artery and vein. In patients who are unconscious, rapid intubation will be required to maintain the airway and prevent aspiration of blood. Conscious patients should lie face-down to maintain a clear airway. Haemorrhage can be controlled initially by applying firm pressure with fingers and thumbs to the free wound margins. Blind application of artery forceps should be avoided if at all possible, lest branches of the facial nerve should be damaged.

If direct pressure is insufficient to control haemorrhage, a naso-gastric tube should be passed and the patient should urgently be taken to the operating theatre, where bleeding vessels can be ligated and the wound can be adequately explored under general anaesthetic.

Wounds to the eyelid margins

Wounds involving the eyelid margin should not be closed in the accident and emergency department, but should be referred to the ophthalmic, plastic, or maxillofacial surgeon. Accurate repair of these wounds is most important, not only for cosmetic reasons but also to avoid the complication of an entropion or ectropion developing secondary to scar contraction on the lower lid, or uneven contact of the upper lid with the eye when blinking. Damage to the upper end of the lacrimal duct may occur in deep wounds of the lower eyelid near the medial canthus. If this is suspected, specialist referral is required.

Injuries to the external ear

The pinna of the external ear consists of convolutions of elastic cartilage covered with adherent skin. Blunt trauma to the pinna often causes a subcutaneous haematoma, which, if not drained, results in deformity (the cauliflower ear). Treatment consists of drainage of the haematoma either by aspiration with a needle or by a small incision under local anaesthetic. The convolutions of the pinna should then be carefully packed (ribbon gauze soaked in thick Iodoform paste is adequate for this purpose) and a pressure bandage should be applied. Follow-up within three days is required, as there is a tendency for seroma formation, and the drainage procedure may need to be repeated.

Straightforward wounds of the pinna with no tissue loss can be repaired by closure with sutures in the usual manner under local anaesthetic. On some occasions there is a considerable amount of skin loss, with exposure of the cartilage (often the result of human bites!). In these circumstances a plastic surgery referral is appropriate, as skin grafting may be required in preference to excision of exposed cartilage, which may lead to considerable deformity of the pinna (Spock ears!).

Some patients who have sustained trauma to the pinna may complain of unilateral deafness secondary to perforation of the tympanic membrane. Auroscopy should be performed to confirm the diagnosis, and a broad-spectrum antibiotic should be prescribed prior to referral to the ENT clinic.

Injury to the facial nerve

The facial nerve (Fig. 3.3) emerges from the base of the skull through the stylomastoid foramen, and, after giving off the posterior auricular nerve, the main nerve then enters the parotid gland, where it gives off its five main branches. From the top down, these are:

1. Temporal branch
This nerve crosses the zygomatic arch, supplying auricularis anterior and superior, and part of frontalis.

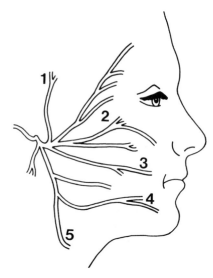

Fig. 3.3 • Diagram illustrating the distribution of the main branches of the facial nerve: 1. temporal; 2. zygomatic; 3. buccal; 4. mandibular; 5. cervical.

2. Zygomatic branches
The branches of this nerve supply frontalis and the upper half of orbicularis oculi. As they cross the zygomatic arch they may be divided as a result of deep wounds at this site, or in fractures of the zygomatic arch. The lower branches supply the lower half of orbicularis oculi and the muscles below the orbit. Some branches pass to both upper and lower lids, and damage to these nerves may result in inability to blink, with subsequent problems of corneal dessication and ulceration.

3. Buccal branch
This nerve supplies the buccinator and the muscle fibres of the upper lip. Damage to this nerve causes paralysis of the upper lip and difficulty in chewing.

4. Mandibular branch
This nerve supplies the muscles of the lower lip. It passes into the neck below the angle of the mandible, and then runs

anteriorly and superiorly across the inferior border of the body of the mandible, where it is particularly at risk from damage from deep wounds, resulting in paralysis of the lower lip.

5. Cervical branch
This nerve passes downwards from the lower border of the parotid gland behind the mandible and supplies the platysma muscle.

Damage to any of the above branches should be suspected with any deep facial wound, and muscle function around the eyes, lips, and cheeks should be tested in the conscious patient. Nerve-repair requires the use of a microscope and the skills of the plastic or maxillofacial surgeon, and immediate consultation with the specialist team is required. Primary nerve-repair is the treatment of choice, and should be performed as soon as possible after the injury has been sustained. Failure to recognize damage to the branches of the facial nerve at the time of the patient's initial presentation reduces the chance of a successful subsequent nerve-repair.

Damage to sensory nerves

Branches of the trigeminal nerve are the sensory nerves to the facial skin, and may be damaged by deep facial wounds. The absence of touch and light pinprick sensation should be recorded before referral to the maxillofacial surgeon. Repair of sensory nerves is not always possible, and a permanent sensory deficit may occur.

Parotid gland and duct

The parotid gland is the largest salivary gland, is wedge-shaped, and lies behind the posterior border of the ascending ramus of the mandible. The superficial lobe extends forward over the masseter muscle, the rest of the gland forming the deep lobe. The parotid duct passes anteriorly across the masseter and then medially at the anterior border of this muscle to pierce the buccinator. It opens on the mucous membrane of the cheek opposite the second upper molar tooth. Both the gland and the duct may be damaged in deep facial wounds in association with branches of the facial nerve, necessitating surgical exploration and repair by the maxillofacial team. Failure to recognize damage to the gland and duct may give rise to the formation of a salivary fistula.

Facial infections

The most commonly encountered infected facial lesions are boils or infected epidermal cysts. These are rarely encountered in hospital practice at an early stage, when antibiotic treatment alone would be expected to be curative. Early treatment is required, as infection may spread via the deep facial vein, resulting in the serious complication of cavernous sinus thrombosis. Incision and drainage is usually required, and general anaesthesia is preferable for large abscesses. A swab should be taken for culture, and then, either the drainage wound should be primarily sutured, or, with a large abscess cavity, a wick soaked in antiseptic solution should be inserted. A 5-day course of flucloxacillin should be prescribed, as the causative organism is most likely to be *Staphylococcus aureus*. If a wick has been inserted into the abscess cavity, delayed skin closure can be undertaken once the cavity is clean. It is important to determine that facial infection is not of dental origin, lest a sinus should be produced when the skin is incised.

Further reading

Eriksson, E. (1979). *Illustrated handbook in local anaesthesia*, 2nd edn. Lloyd Luke, London.

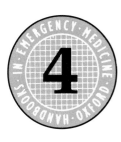

CHAPTER 4

Initial assessment and management of maxillofacial trauma

Key points in initial assessment and management of maxillofacial trauma

1 Maxillofacial trauma is rarely immediately life-threatening unless there is a compromised airway or major haemorrhage.

2 Cervical spinal injury should be assumed in any patient who has sustained major injury above the level of the clavicle.

3 Facial injuries may be associated with skull fractures and intracranial complication.

4 In the context of multiple injuries, once a clear airway has been established, repair of the facial component should not precede any surgical procedure required for intra-abdominal, intrathoracic, or intracranial injury, and patients must be adequately resuscitated initially.

5 Most fractures of the facial skeleton can be diagnosed on clinical examination. Radiological examination will determine the extent of fractures and assist the maxillofacial surgeon in planning the appropriate surgical procedure.

Introduction

It is important to assess priorities in the initial management of injured patients, especially in those with multiple injuries. Facial injuries only need immediate treatment if the airway is at risk or there is major bleeding. It is dangerous to transfer a patient with facial injuries to the maxillofacial surgeons if life-threatening injuries in the chest or abdomen have not been recognized and treated. A systematic approach is needed to diagnose life-threatening injuries. The first section of this chapter concerns priorities in the management of patients with multiple injuries. The second section deals specifically with examination of facial injuries.

Assessment of the multiply-injured patient

- **Airway control   Respiratory difficulties   Shock
  Neurological status   Priorities for surgical intervention**

Multiply-injured patients should be assessed at an early stage by experienced senior doctors. In many hospitals there is a trauma team specifically for this purpose. The patient should initially be admitted to a brightly-lit and well-equipped resuscitation room, preferably with an adjacent emergency operating theatre. A clear history of the accident should be obtained from the ambulance personnel. Details should include the time, place, and circumstances of the accident, the initial assessment of injuries sustained, what treatment has been initiated, and whether there has been any change in the patient's condition, especially in pulse and conscious level. A primary survey should be carried out rapidly to assess airway patency and adequacy of respiration and to detect shock.

Airway control

A patent airway is essential. A patient who can talk normally must have a patent airway; but any abnormal phonation or snoring indicates a partially obstructed airway. In an unconscious patient the airway is always at risk. All patients who are unconscious or who have major blunt injury above the clavicle must be assumed to have an injury to the cervical spine: the neck should be supported by a stiff collar and sandbags until a lateral X-ray of the cervical spine has shown no fracture or dislocation.

The airway is likely to be compromised under several circumstances:

In an unconscious patient the tongue may have fallen back, obstructing the oropharynx. If an unstable neck injury has not been excluded, this form of obstruction can be relieved by lifting the mandible forwards by the chin-lift or jaw-thrust manœuvres and the insertion of an oral airway. The tongue may be displaced backwards in association with bilateral fractures of the body or symphysis of the mandible. Patency of the airway can then be restored by pulling the fractured segment forwards, or by inserting a mattress suture or a towel clip through the tongue and applying gentle forward traction.

Occasionally a fractured maxilla is displaced backwards enough to compromise the airway by contact between the soft palate and the posterior pharyngeal wall. The airway obstruction can be relieved by pulling the maxilla forwards and upwards, with two fingers hooked up behind the hard palate.

Foreign bodies, detached tooth fragments, and vomit should be removed by gentle sweeping movements with the partially flexed index finger or by the use of McGill forceps and suction. Any missing teeth should be noted, as they may have been inhaled, and should be looked for on a chest X-ray (Fig. 4.1). Broken dentures or avulsed teeth should be kept, as subsequent reconstitution of a whole denture or tooth may rule out the possibility of inhaled fragments.

Blood may accumulate rapidly in the pharynx after fractures of the facial bones or the base of the skull. There may also be bleeding from wounds of the tongue and mouth. A rigid large-bore sucker (Yankauer) should be used to remove blood. Fine-bore catheters should be used only through an endotracheal or naso-pharyngeal tube. It may be possible to

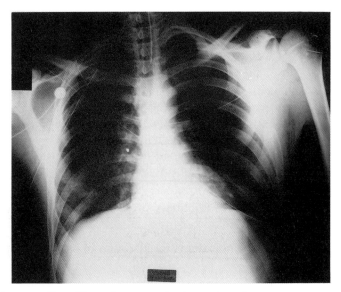

Fig. 4.1 • Chest X-ray, demonstrating inhalation of amalgam into the right bronchial tree.

clip off a bleeding vessel under direct vision; but, more often than not, no bleeding-point is visible, particularly if there are facial fractures. Anterior or posterior nasal packing will reduce bleeding from the ethmoidal arteries. For this purpose either epistaxis catheters or size 12–14 Foley catheters are lubricated and passed through the nostrils into the post-nasal space. The balloons are filled with air, and anterior traction is applied until the balloon occludes the choana. An anterior balloon, if present, can then be inflated within the nostril, or alternatively, the nose can be packed with ribbon gauze. The passage of two naso-pharyngeal airways will also assist in reducing epistaxis when there is difficulty in maintaining an adequate oral airway. A safety-pin should be inserted through the end of each tube to prevent backward displacement. If, despite these measures and the appropriate packing and direct pressure on readily accessible wounds, haemorrhage into the airway persists, endotracheal intubation should be attempted by a competent operator, minimizing movements of the cervical spine, which should be stabilized by an assistant's firmly holding the patient's head in a neutral position.

There may be direct trauma to the airway. This should be suspected if there is bruising and swelling of the front of the neck, with subcutaneous emphysema. There may be abnormal mobility of the larynx. Laryngeal injury should also be suspected on detecting abnormal phonation. Despite the damage to the airway, it may be possible for an experienced anaesthetist to pass an endotracheal tube; but, if this is not possible, a cricothyroidotomy, or rarely a tracheostomy, will be needed.

Endotracheal intubation

Box 4.1 **Indications for insertion of an endotracheal tube**

- Absent gag reflex with doubtful airway
- Grossly impacted maxilla which resists advancement
- Profuse post-nasal haemorrhage
- Major head injury
- Associated chest injuries, for example flail chest

It is important to stress that endotracheal intubation is a difficult procedure in patients with major maxillofacial trauma, and should only be performed by someone experienced in this technique, usually a senior anaesthetist. Anaesthetic and paralysing agents will usually be required. Oral endotracheal intubation is preferred to nasal intubation, especially if a fracture of the skull base is suspected or if there is rhinorrhoea. As has been previously mentioned, the presence of a cervical spinal injury makes endotracheal intubation extremely hazardous, and cricothyroidotomy may be preferable.

Cricothyroidotomy
Cricothyroidotomy is indicated when attempts to intubate the trachea have failed.

Surgical cricothyroidotomy After sterilizing the skin and injecting 1 to 2 ml of local anaesthetic subcutaneously, the thyroid cartilage is stabilized with the fingers and thumb of one hand while a 2 cm transverse incision is made over the cricothyroid membrane, which in turn is divided to allow the insertion of a cuffed tracheostomy tube. The cuff is inflated and the tube is secured in position by tying the attached tapes. In children the cricoid cartilage is the only circumferential support to the upper trachea, and surgical cricothyroidotomy is therefore not recommended in children under 12 years of age.

Needle cricothyroidotomy In cases *in extremis* and in children, needle cricothyroidotomy can be performed. Having sterilized the skin, a size 12 needle with an overlying cannula is attached to a 5 or 10 ml syringe, and the needle is introduced through the cricothyroid membrane while angled caudally at 45 degrees. The syringe should be gently aspirated as the needle is advanced. Free aspiration of air demonstrates that the needle is in the airway. The cannula is then advanced and the needle removed. The stem of a T paediatric endotracheal tube connector is attached to the cannula via a short length of oxygen tubing (Fig. 4.2). One of the T connectors is attached to oxygen tubing, and the oxygen flow is adjusted to a rate of 15 litres per minute. Ventilation is controlled by the thumb's being placed over the free end of the T connector in a sequence of inspiration (thumb on for one second) and expiration (thumb removed for 4 seconds). This technique should only be used for about 30 minutes before a surgical cricothyroidotomy or tracheostomy is performed. Prolonged use of jet insufflation of oxygen through a small cannula inevitably leads to carbon dioxide retention.

Emphasis has been placed, thus far, on maintenance of an airway in patients who may have a cervical spinal injury or other injuries in which movement is contraindicated. In isolated major facial injuries or where injury to the cervical spine has been confidently excluded, the airway can be maintained by placing the patient in the recovery position on a trolley tilted head-down. This enables blood, saliva, and vomit to escape through the mouth or to be removed by means of a sucker.

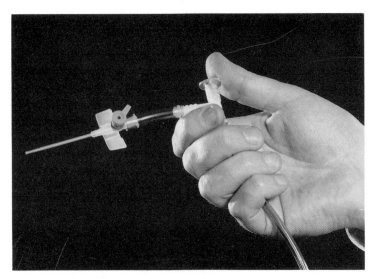

Fig. 4.2 • Demonstration of oxygen tubing circuit connected to an intravenous cannula used following needle cricothyroidotomy.

Respiratory difficulties

When the airway is patent and secure, the adequacy and rate of respiration should be noted. Inspection may reveal cyanosis, bruising to the chest wall, open chest wounds, unequal chest movement, or paradoxical respiration associated with a flail chest. The trachea should be palpated in the suprasternal notch to detect any deviation suggesting mediastinal shift. Palpation of the chest wall may reveal subcutaneous emphysema. Auscultation may reveal decreased air entry or absent breath sounds, indicating pneumothorax, haemothorax, or pulmonary contusion. On clinical suspicion of a tension pneumothorax, a large-bore needle should be immediately inserted into the second intercostal space lateral to the mid-clavicular line. This should be left in position until a chest drain is inserted, normally in the fifth intercostal space anterior to the mid-axillary line. A chest X-ray should then be obtained, preferably in an erect or semi-erect position if the patient's condition permits.

Arterial blood-gas analysis should be carried out, and all patients should receive oxygen in high concentration, i.e. more than 80 per cent.

Shock

Hypovolaemia is not a feature associated with head injury, and is rarely a consequence of facial injury. If a patient with facial injury is shocked, one should therefore look elsewhere, especially for intrathoracic or intra-abdominal bleeding, or pelvic fractures. Decreased capillary refill, following the application of pressure on the fingernail, is a simple yet useful test of the adequacy of the circulation. The presence of skin pallor, tachycardia, and tachypnoea should be noted. Hypotension in young and middle-aged adults suggests a loss of at least 30 per cent of blood volume, and is an ominous sign. Two large intravenous cannulae should be inserted, if possible, into the anterior cubital veins. If upper-limb access is not possible due to injury, a cut-down should be performed on the long saphenous veins. Blood should be withdrawn for haemoglobin estimation and for cross-matching. Urea and electrolytes estimation preoperatively may be of some value in the elderly and for those patients on diuretics.

Traumatic shock should be treated aggressively with rapid infusion of colloid or crystalloid solutions. Transfusion of group O rhesus negative blood may be required until fully cross-matched blood is available. Iatrogenic fluid overload is uncommon in post-traumatic haemorrhagic shock, but haemodynamic measurements should be carefully monitored, especially in the elderly and in children. While limb fractures can usually be detected clinically, peritoneal lavage or abdominal ultrasound may be required to demonstrate blood loss into the peritoneal cavity. Pulse-rate, blood-pressure, central venous pressure, and urinary output should be constantly monitored during resuscitation.

Neurological status

Many patients with major maxillofacial trauma have also sustained cranial and intracranial injury. The patient's conscious level should be assessed according to the Glasgow

Coma Scale. Secondary brain insults due to hypoxia and hypovolaemia should be corrected by the administration of oxygen in high concentration and infusion of intravenous fluids. Some patients may be intoxicated; but a decrease in conscious level should not automatically be attributed solely to the effects of alcohol. Bleeding and CSF leakage from nose and ears should be noted. Scalp wounds should be inspected and palpated gently with a gloved finger to detect any underlying fracture. Bleeding scalp vessels should be ligated. Pupil size and reaction to light should be assessed, and the eye should be carefully examined for any evidence of direct injury (see p. 64).

Once a patent airway has been established, the stomach should be emptied by a gastric tube, which should be passed through the mouth rather than the nose if there are major maxillary fractures or a basal skull fracture is suspected. Once resuscitation is well under way, X-rays of the skull should be performed or, if appropriate, a CT scan should be arranged.

Priorities for surgical intervention

When the airway and breathing are adequate and fluid replacement is under way, the next priority is to stop any major bleeding within the abdomen or chest. Essential neurosurgical procedures should be performed next. Certain orthopaedic procedures, such as fixation of an unstable spinal injury or external fixation of major pelvic fractures, also require a degree of urgency. These operations would normally take precedence over maxillofacial surgery, although it may be possible for two surgical teams to work at the same time.

General examination of the injured face

- **Fractures to the maxilla and zygoma Eye injuries Nasal injuries The mandible Radiological examination Specialist referral**

After life-threatening injuries have been diagnosed and resuscitative procedures have been instigated, a more detailed assessment of any maxillofacial injury should be made. A similar approach is needed in patients who have only facial injuries.

Many facial injuries have important medico-legal implications, as they are often caused by assault, road-traffic accidents, or accidents at work. Obtaining a clear history may be difficult if the patient is intoxicated or has been unconscious. In children the possibility of non-accidental injury should always be considered.

The injuries should be examined by inspection and palpation, followed by appropriate radiological examination.

Fractures to the maxilla and zygoma

The face should be inspected from in front, in side profile, and also from above by standing behind the patient to assess any asymmetry. Flattening of the cheek is a sign of a depressed zygomatic fracture. A 'dish face' deformity occurs when there is posterior displacement of the maxilla secondary to major fracture. Any deformity of the nose should be noted. The position and distribution of bruising of the skin and soft-tissue swelling should be noted. The bones should be palpated to elicit tenderness, crepitus, or depression. A depressed fracture of the zygomatic arch is usually detectable on palpation. The zygomatico-frontal suture on the lateral aspect of the orbit and the zygomatico-maxillary suture below the orbit should be palpated for tenderness. These sutures are often disrupted in displaced zygomatic fractures. A 'step' may be palpable in fractures involving the infraorbital margin. Injury to the infraorbital nerve at the infraorbital foramen results in hypoaesthesia of the cheek, the side of the nose, and the upper lip. Any loss of skin sensation can be tested by stroking both cheeks with the fingertips. Numbness of the upper incisor, canine, and premolar teeth indicates damage to the anterior superior alveolar nerve where it branches from the infraorbital nerve in the infraorbital canal. The presence of subcutaneous emphysema indicates a fracture into a sinus, usually the maxillary. The patient should be advised not to blow the nose, as this will force air through the fracture into the soft tissues or the orbit. Fractures extending into the air sinuses are compound fractures, and antibiotics, for example Augmentin 375 mg three times a day should be prescribed. Following clinical examination, appropriate facial bone X-rays should be ordered to confirm the injuries (see Box 4.2).

Eye injuries

The eye is commonly injured in association with facial trauma (Fig. 4.3). In addition to a history of the present injury, it is important to know about any previous ophthalmic surgery or any eye disease requiring medication. Once an adequate history has been obtained, the eye should be carefully examined.

Periorbital swelling may develop quickly, and it is important to assess the eye before separation of the eyelids becomes impossible. Even when swelling has developed, it is important to separate the eyelids to examine the eye. In conscious patients some attempt should be made to assess visual acuity, even if this is only a relatively crude test, such as counting the number of fingers held 3 feet away from the patient. Assessment of any visual-field defect should also be made. Contact lenses should be removed immediately after visual acuity has been tested.

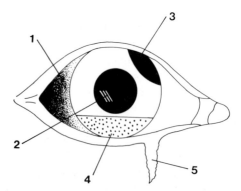

Fig. 4.3 • Diagram of the eye to show some features of injury:
1. subconjunctival haemorrhage with no posterior border, indicative of an orbital fracture; 2. corneal abrasion; 3. iridodialysis; 4. hyphaema;
5. wound extending through the lower eyelid margin.

Traumatic exophthalmos indicates a retrobulbar haemorrhage with increased intra-orbital pressure. This may compromise the blood-supply to the retina and optic nerve, and result in blindness. Urgent referral to an ophthalmologist is essential.

Enophthalmos may result from fractures of the floor of the orbit with herniation of intraorbital contents. It may also be noted that the pupils are on different horizontal planes. The distance between the eyes may be widened (traumatic telecanthus) by a severe naso-ethmoidal fracture.

Diplopia, especially on vertical gaze, may occur with fractures of the orbital floor and oedema or trapping of the inferior rectus and inferior oblique muscles. This is often temporary, but if it persists indicates tethering of the muscle in the fracture. Other causes of diplopia should also be considered, for example, damage to III, IV, and VI cranial nerves following a head injury.

Pupil size and reaction to light should be noted. In the presence of an intracranial haematoma, a dilated pupil is almost always on the same side as the haematoma. A dilated pupil which does not respond to light is a late sign of cerebral compression, and bilateral fixed dilated pupils indicate very severe brain dysfunction. A dilated pupil may result from direct trauma to the eye. This is called traumatic mydriasis, and is thought to be caused by interference with the ciliary nerves due to temporary distortion of the eyeball at the time of impact. Although normally a transient phenomenon, it may result in permanent pupil dilatation. Distortion of the pupil can result from a tear in the iris sphincter. Peripheral detachment of the iris (iridodialysis) may cause a visual-field defect, and surgical repair may be required.

With the head in the erect position a hyphaema may be seen as a fluid level in the anterior chamber. Blood in the anterior chamber of a supine patient results in loss of the red reflex normally seen through the ophthalmoscope, and the fundus cannot be seen. Ophthalmic referral is required.

The anterior surface of the eye should be closely examined for any perforating injury. The presence of intraocular foreign bodies should be considered, and appropriate orbital X-rays should be taken if necessary. If a perforation of the eye is demonstrated, no drops should be instilled, but an eye-patch should be applied and the patient should be referred to the ophthalmologist. In the absence of any perforating injury, foreign bodies on the surface of the eye should be removed after instilling amethocaine eye-drops as necessary. Corneal abrasions can be demonstrated by the use of fluorescein drops.

Subconjunctival haemorrhage is common following a blow to the eye. If a posterior limit can be located, this indicates local injury to the eye; but if no posterior limit is visible the diagnosis is a fracture of the orbital wall.

The fundus of the eye should be examined with an ophthalmoscope. This may show papilloedema or injuries such as retinal tears or detachment, vitreous haemorrhage, or dislocation of the lens. This latter condition results in gross impairment of visual acuity.

Wounds of the eyelids should be closely examined. A full-thickness wound should raise suspicion of an underlying penetrating injury of the eye. Wounds which traverse the eyelid margin require specialist repair. The most serious site for these wounds is at the medial end of the lower eyelid where the lower lacrimal canaliculus may be involved, resulting in overflow of tears on to the face. This clinical feature may also be noted if there is any damage to the naso-lacrimal duct.

Nasal injuries

The nose, as the most prominent part of the face, is injured frequently. It is helpful to know about any previous nasal trauma. An obvious nasal deformity in an assaulted patient may result from a previous battle! Crepitus or abnormal mobility may be elicited on palpation of the nasal bones. The nasal airways should be inspected for septal deviation or a septal haematoma requiring surgical drainage. In addition to epistaxis there may be leakage of cerebro-spinal fluid, indicating a fracture through the cribriform plate of the ethmoid bone. There is then a danger of meningitis, and prophylactic antibiotics such as augmentin or amoxycillin should be prescribed.

Traumatic epistaxis may be severe, with consequent

swallowing and later vomiting of blood. Nasal bleeding which cannot be controlled by packs should be treated by inserting an epistaxis catheter to control bleeding from branches of the anterior ethmoidal artery. Blood should be cross-matched, and an intravenous infusion should be commenced as a preliminary to urgent referral to the maxillofacial or ENT surgeon.

Displaced fractures are usually obvious clinically, and undisplaced fractures do not require any specific treatment. Radiological demonstration of a fracture may be important for medico-legal purposes, but it is often difficult for the radiologist to state with confidence whether a fracture of the nasal bones is recent or old. Manipulation of the nose following fracture of the bones or displacement of the cartilaginous septum is indicated to restore an obstructed nasal airway or for cosmetic purposes. Opinions vary as to exactly when manipulation should be performed, but it should certainly not be delayed for more than ten days from the time of injury. Manipulation after this time becomes increasingly difficult, and an elective rhinoplasty at a later date may be required.

The mandible

The patient should be asked about the site of pain, any malocclusion, and any loose or missing teeth. Any soft-tissue swelling should be noted on external inspection, and the mandible should be gently palpated for tenderness and the presence of a 'step', indicating an underlying fracture. With unstable fractures there may be obvious deformity. The mandible is often fractured at a site distant from the point of impact, for example a fall on the chin may cause condylar or subcondylar fractures. Bleeding from the external auditory meatus may be associated with fractures of the coronoid fossa. Inability to close the mouth occurs with temporomandibular joint dislocation. The mouth should be inspected for malaligned, fractured, or missing teeth, and for haemorrhage due to a compound fracture. A mandibular fracture may cause bruising of overlying mucosa or a sublingual haematoma. The tongue should be inspected for any wound or bleeding.

Radiological examination

X-rays of the facial bones are necessary to confirm the diagnosis and to assist the maxillofacial surgeon in planning appropriate treatment of facial fractures.

Box 4.2 X-rays which assist in the diagnosis of maxillofacial injury

- 30° and 45° occipitomental views
- Lateral facial bone view

These standard X-rays are often referred to as 'facial views' and show fractures of the maxilla and zygoma.

- Submental vertical — shows fractures of the zygomatic arch.
- PA and lateral oblique views / Orthopantomogram — Show fractures of the mandible.
- Occipito-mental and lateral views demonstrate fractures of the nasal bones and septal deviation.
- Tomography — sometimes required to demonstrate fractures of the orbital floor. This is normally arranged by the maxillofacial surgeon.
- CT scanning — may more accurately delineate the extent of major facial fractures and associated fractures at the base of the skull and in the cervical spine.

Interpretation of X-rays of the facial skeleton and skull always poses a problem for the relatively inexperienced doctor in the accident department. It is important that adequate teaching should be provided to ensure that important landmarks of the facial skeleton and features of fractures can be readily recognized. Good-quality X-rays are essential, and require the co-operation of the patient. Films of diagnostic quality are unlikely to be achieved in patients who are intoxicated with alcohol or restless for other reasons, for example, from hypoxia, shock, or the effect of drugs. Often X-ray examination can be deferred for several hours until the patient can hold the head still.

In patients with multiple injuries, radiological examination of the facial bones is much less important than X-rays of the cervical spine, chest, skull, and pelvis. If the neck is immobilized it will not be possible to obtain standard facial bone X-rays, although a lateral view of the skull in the supine patient may demonstrate fluid levels in the sinuses due to fractures of the sinus walls. Tomography is sometimes used in the diagnosis of a fracture of the orbital floor; but there is no urgency about this.

CT scanning, if readily available, can give more information about the exact site and extent of fractures of the facial skeleton, skull, and cervical spine. This investigation should only be carried out once hypovolaemia and hypoxia have been corrected and the airway is secured, if necessary by anaesthesia, endotracheal intubation, and ventilation.

Box 4.3 Other important radiological investigations

Cervical spine
- Lateral C1 to C7/T1
- Antero-posterior
- Transoral view of odontoid process

Chest

Skull
- P/A
- Lateral
- Townes

In addition to radiological examination to confirm the presence of fractures of the facial skeleton, X-rays of the cervical spine, skull, and chest are often necessary. The most useful film of the cervical spine is the lateral view, and it should be stressed that the articulation of C7/T1 must be demonstrated. Often this can only be achieved by pulling the patient's arms to move the shoulders down. If this fails, a transaxillary ('swimmer's') view should be taken.

Plain films will usually demonstrate any fracture of the vault of the skull. Basal fractures cannot normally be seen, owing to the thickness of the bone; but a fluid level in the sphenoidal sinus is indicative of a basal fracture, as is an anterior aerocoele seen on the 'brow-up' lateral view.

Chest radiography is essential in multiply-injured patients, and may show fractured ribs, pneumothorax, haemothorax, pulmonary contusion, aspiration pneumonia, or widening of the mediastinum. Where the patient's condition permits, an erect or semi-erect film gives more information than a film taken in the supine position. Chest X-ray will also demonstrate the position of an endotracheal tube and a central venous monitoring catheter. In the context of the maxillofacial injury, chest X-ray may also demonstrate the presence of inhaled teeth.

Specialist referral

In hospitals with a maxillofacial and oral surgical department, a specialist opinion can be rapidly obtained when required. However, there is no such department in many district general hospitals, and on-site specialist opinions are not immediately available. The nearest maxillofacial department should provide clear guidelines to the accident and emergency staff about the priorities for referral. A telephone conversation describing the nature of the injury will normally enable appropriate action to be taken. Many injuries are sustained at night, and patients can often be admitted under observation in the referring hospital and transferred to the maxillofacial unit the following day. Urgent referral is normally required in the following circumstances:

1. Major fractures of the maxilla (Le Fort). If the airway is at risk, the patient should be anaesthetized and intubated before transfer and accompanied by an anaesthetist. The patient should be adequately resuscitated, and other more urgent injuries, such as splenic rupture, should have been dealt with by the surgical team in the referring hospital before transfer.

2. Displaced and unstable mandibular fractures.

3. Where there is difficulty in controlling major haemorrhage and transfer would be hazardous, the maxillofacial surgeon should attend the patient in the referring hospital.

4. Avulsed teeth that cannot be adequately replaced in their sockets.

5. Bleeding from a tooth socket following extraction that cannot be adequately controlled.

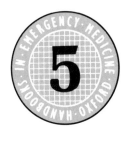

CHAPTER 5

Assessment and management of mandibular fractures and dislocations of the temporomandibular joint

Key points in mandibular trauma

1 The majority of mandibular fractures are caused by interpersonal assaults.
2 The neck and body of the mandible are the common sites of fracture in mandibular trauma.
3 Most mandibular fractures are compound, and therefore require prompt treatment and prophylatic antibiotics.
4 Sublingual haematoma, paraesthesia (or anaesthesia) of the lower lip, and derangement of occlusion are important clinical features of mandibular trauma.
5 Orthopantomograms and/or lateral oblique mandibular X-rays and posterior anterior mandibular X-rays are very helpful in diagnosis, but radiographic evaluation is only secondary to systematic clinical examination.
6 Most temporomandibular dislocations can be effectively treated in casualty by giving intravenous diazepam and physically manipulating the jaw into position.

Basic anatomy

The mandible occupies and forms the lower part of the face, and articulates with the mandibular fossa of the skull (Fig. 5.1).

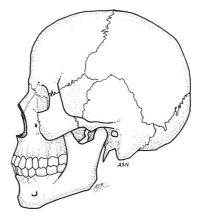

Fig. 5.1 • Mandible in articulation with skull.

Aetiology

There are many possible causes of mandibular fracture, the most common being:

(1) road-traffic accidents;

(2) assaults;

(3) sports injuries;

(4) falls;

(5) industrial accidents; and

(6) others (for example, pathological fractures due to neoplasms, infections, etc).

Sites of fracture

The site of fracture can be influenced by local factors such as mandibular atrophy due to ridge resorption, unerupted teeth, or pathology, for example, cysts, neoplasms, etc. The most common sites in order of occurrence are (Fig. 5.2):

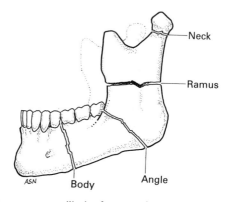

Fig. 5.2 • Common mandibular fracture sites.

(1) the neck of the mandible
(2) the body of the mandible
(3) the angle; and
(4) the ramus.

Often there is more than one fracture, so after finding one look for others.

Signs and symptoms

1. Pain
2. Swelling (Fig. 5.3)
3. Bleeding

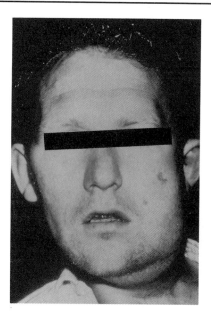

Fig. 5.3 • Facial swelling associated with fractured mandible.

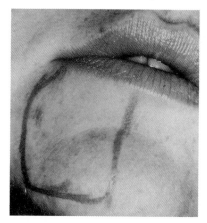

Fig. 5.4 • Mental nerve anaesthesia to show region of anaesthesia when mandibular fracture involves alveolar nerve.

4. Paraesthesia (anaesthesia of the lower lip) (Fig. 5.4)
5. Buccal haematoma (Fig. 5.5)
6. Sublingual haematoma
7. Extraoral haematoma
8. Avulsed teeth (Fig. 5.6)

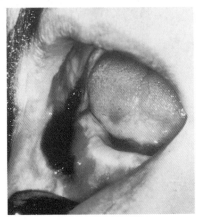

Fig. 5.5 • Intraoral buccal haematoma associated with mandibular fracture.

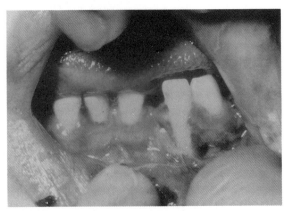

Fig. 5.6 • Displacement of tooth at site of fracture.

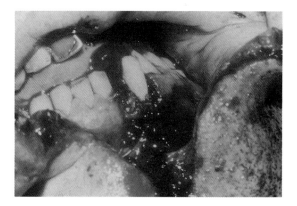

Fig. 5.7 • Occlusal derangement with step displacement of mandibular fracture.

9. Derangement of occlusion (Fig. 5.7), which can result in:
   (a) anterior open bite;
   (b) loss of occlusion unilaterally; and
   (c) deviation of the mandible.
10. Difficulty with swallowing, breathing, and speech
11. Mobility of the fracture
12. Deformity
13. Non-fit of dentures

Clinical examination and general management

• **Extraoral examination   Intraoral examination**

The aim of any treatment is to preserve life, maintain function, and restore appearance. It is essential to do a proper general and local examination of the patient to exclude any other serious injury, to check the level of consciousness, and to see whether there is any cerebral damage and haemorrhage present.

Box 5.1 General management

- Preservation of airway and breathing
- Arrest of haemorrhage and replacement of IV fluids/ Blood if necessary
- Control of pain
- Prevention of infection

Once a proper general assessment has been made of the patient a local examination of the fracture site is made. This is made easier if the blood, mud, debris, etc. is cleared from the face and intra-orally. This simple cleaning helps the local assessment greatly. Another help is cleaning the wound itself, as it aids visualization. Once removal of gross debris and toilet of the wound is complete, a detailed examination of the fracture site can be made both extra-and intra-orally.

Box 5.2 Local treatment

- Remove gross debris
- Toilet of wound
- Detailed examination and assessment of injury

Assessment of fractures should include:

(1) position of fracture(s);

(2) displacement of fracture(s);

(3) soft-tissue condition (antitetanus required?);

(4) teeth available; and

(5) associated conditions—medical or other conditions.

Extraoral examination

The patient is examined for any bruising and swelling, as these give an indication of the site of fracture. It is important to palpate the swelling gently to check for any bony defects underneath which may be masked. A general palpation of the lower border of the mandible is also made to check for any crepitus, steps, or breaks in the mandible. It is also important to assess the patient for any anaesthesia/paraesthesia that may be present in the lower lip/chin region. On completion of the extraoral examination an intraoral examination is then made.

Intraoral examination

In order to do this properly it is best to be systematic in your approach, examining the soft tissue, teeth, and hard tissue in that order.

Soft-tissue examination

Check for any buccal and lingual haematoma or bleeding, making a special note if there is any sublingual haematoma present, since this is almost pathognomonic of mandibular fractures. It is important to note any soft-tissue injury, especially injuries involving the tongue or communicating directly with the fracture (Figs 5.5 and 5.7).

Examination of teeth and occlusion

It is vital to check for any missing teeth, fragments of teeth, or fractured restorations, as these may easily have been inhaled by the patient, especially if he or she has been unconscious. A chest radiograph is essential under these circumstances. The teeth should be tested for excess mobility, as they may be dislodged and inhaled. If the patient is edentulous and has dentures these must be removed and put in a safe place, as they might be needed later for making gunning splints to treat the patient. Step defects in the occlusal plane give an indication of the fracture site. If no steps are present the fracture site can be located in most cases by gentle palpation. The fractures can be classified as being favourable or unfavourable in the vertical and horizontal directions. The displacement and stability of a fracture depends on whether it is vertically and horizontally favourable or unfavourable. A favourable fracture is one in which the muscles hold the fracture-ends together, thereby maintaining stability and aiding healing (Fig. 5.8a,b). An unfavourable

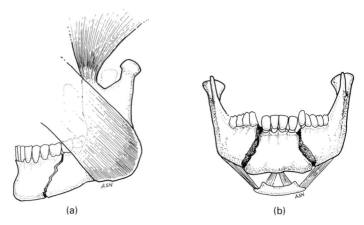

(a)   (b)

Fig. 5.8 • Diagrams demonstrating a favourable fracture of the mandible. (a) Lateral; (b) frontal.

fracture is one where the muscles cause the fragments to separate or override. This results in instability and non-union of the fracture (Fig. 5.9a,b).

Radiology

To assess the extent of mandibular fractures and their sites, good and relevant radiographs are essential. The radiographs that can be taken to assess mandibular fractures are:

1. *Intraoral*, to assess involvement of teeth in the fracture. These views are however rarely available in Accident and Emergency.

2. *Right and left lateral oblique(s)* show body, angle, ramus, and condyle. These views are needed if there is no orthopantomogram facility present (Fig. 5.10).

3. *Postero-anterior (PA) mandible* (Fig. 5.11) shows fractures of body and angle and the type of displacement present. If angled at 30° the condyles are clear of the mastoid process — this is called the **reverse Towne's view**.

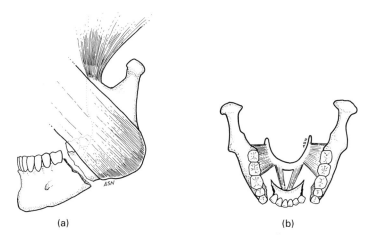

(a)   (b)

Fig. 5.9 • Diagrams demonstrating an unfavourable fracture of the mandible. (a) Lateral; (b) from above.

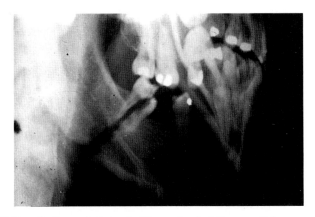

Fig. 5.10 • Radiograph (lateral oblique view) of the mandible.

4. *Orthopantomogram (OPG/OPT)* — a very good view, showing virtually all sites of fracture (Fig. 5.12).
5. *Lower oblique occlusal* shows the degree of displacement present (Fig. 5.13).

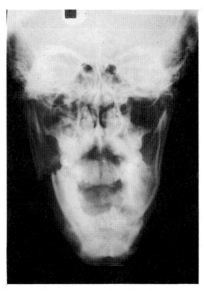

Fig. 5.11 • Radiograph (postero-anterior view) of the mandible.

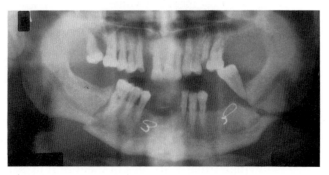

Fig. 5.12 • Radiograph (orthopantomogram: OPG/OPT) of the mandible.

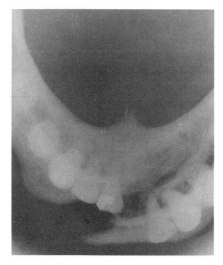

Fig. 5.13 • Radiograph (oblique occlusal view) of the mandible.

Treatment

- **Reduction   Immobilization   Treatment of fractures in children   Postoperative care**

Once assessment is complete the basic treatment plan is:

- reduction;
- fixation; and
- immobilization.

Reduction

Reduction can be carried out under general anaesthesia or local anaesthesia, depending on the severity, the site, and the displacement of the fractures. The teeth are used wherever possible to reduce a fracture to its correct position. If teeth are in the fracture line they can potentially impede healing, because the fracture is compounded into the mouth via the periodontal membrane. If these involved teeth are to be left *in situ* then antibiotics must be given: benzyl penicillin, 600 mg mega unit IV/IM 6-hourly for 2 days, followed by oral penicillin and metronidazole for 7 days. Erythromycin is substituted for penicillin in cases of penicillin allergy.

Immobilization

Immobilization allows bone healing to occur.

The period of immobilization depends on:

- the site of the fracture;
- the age of the patient;
- the presence of teeth; and
- the presence of infection.

Normally, immobilization is needed for a period of 4–6 weeks. However, with the advent of plating as a means of treating fractures immobilization is unnecessary in many cases.

Types of immobilization for mandibular fracture depend on whether the patient is dentate, partially dentate, or edentulous (has no teeth), and whether there are other injuries involving the head, neck, and maxilla. Below is a summary of the approaches and methods currently used:

1. plating (Fig. 5.14a,b);
2. eyelet wiring and intermaxillary fixation (Fig. 5.15);
3. archbars and intermaxillary fixation;
4. Direct bone wires
   (a) upper-border wires;
   (b) lower border wires);
5. pin fixation;
6. intermedullary pins; and
7. bone clamps.

In an edentulous patient gunning splints may be made by modifying the patient's dentures. These are fixed to the upper jaw by perialveolar wires, and to the lower jaw by circumferential wires. The front teeth of the denture are

(a)

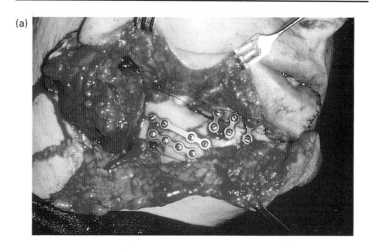

(b)

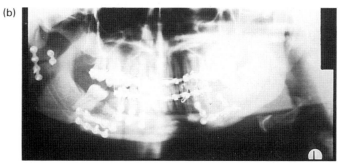

Fig. 5.14 • (a) Reduction of a comminuted fractured mandible through a wound with multiple titanium bone-plates. (b) Radiographic view.

removed to give a gap through which the patient can feed. Hooks to the buccal surface of the denture flanges allow for intermaxillary fixation by elastics or wires.

Treatment of fractures in children

Immobilization is achieved by gunning or McClennan's splints or by use of orthodontic brackets cemented on to teeth. Transosseous fixation or plating is contraindicated in many cases, as it may damage developing tooth germs.

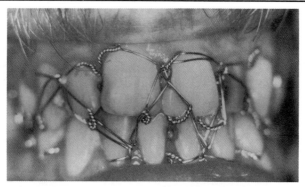

Fig. 5.15 • Reduction of a fractured mandible with eyelet wiring and intermaxillary fixation.

Postoperative care

There are three phases:

- immediate—recovery from general anaesthetic;
- intermediate—during immobilization; and
- late—long-term.

Immediate Postoperative care

- Usual nursing care after a general anaesthetic.
- Essential to have wire cutters, scissors, etc., close to bedside in case of emergency if jaws have been wired.

Intermediate care

Analgesics There is rarely much pain, and analgesics are not required as a routine. Narcotic analgesics such as morphine are contraindicated, as they depress respiratory centres and the cough reflex, and this is dangerous, especially if the patient's consciousness was affected. If sedation is needed 5 mg diazepam may be given IV. Diclofenac (Voltarol) can be used for analgesia, since it can be given IM.

Antibiotics A 5-day course of penicillin in almost all bony injuries. Erythromycin in cases of penicillin allergy.

Oral hygiene Chlorhexidine mouth-washes.

Diet Liquid/semi-solid diet is suggested, particularly if intermaxillary fixation is present.
Fluid balance must be maintained.

Condylar fractures

- **Unilateral   Bilateral**

In cases of *condylar fractures* treatment depends on whether the fractures are unilateral or bilateral, and whether there is any deviation and disturbance of occlusion.

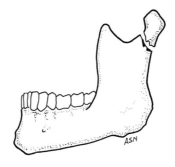

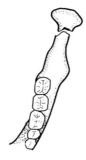

Fig. 5.16 • Diagram demonstrating extracapsular fracture of the mandibular condyle.

Unilateral fractures of the condyle (Fig 5.16)

1. If there are no symptoms and there is no derangement of occlusion then no active treatment is required. It is best to advise the patient to be on a soft diet for up to 2 weeks and to do gentle jaw exercises during this period, to prevent stiffness of the temporomandibular joint.

2. If occlusion is deranged or the jaw deviates to the side of the fracture on opening, then it is best to apply intermaxillary fixation for a period of no more than 2 weeks, as periods longer than this may cause jaw stiffening, and possibly ankylosis of the temporomandibular joint.

Bilateral fractures of the condyle (Fig. 5.17)

All bilateral fractures of the condyle require intermaxillary fixation for a period of 2 weeks minimum.

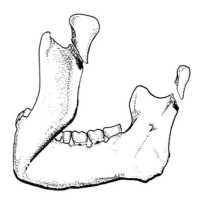

Fig. 5.17 • Bilateral mandibular condylar fractures.

Dislocations of the temporomandibular joint

The condyle of the mandible rests in the glenoid fossa (Fig. 5.18). Dislocation results when the condylar head is displaced out of the glenoid fossa, but still remains within the capsule. Dislocations of the temporomandibular joint (TMJ) are almost always anterior, beyond the articular eminence, and can be bilateral or unilateral (Fig. 5.19).

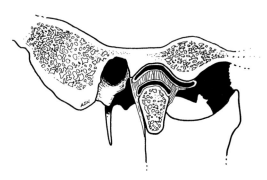

Fig. 5.18 • Anatomy of the temporomandibular joint.

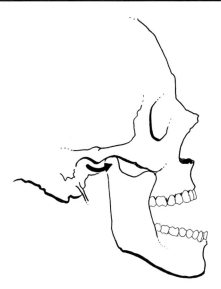

Fig. 5.19 • Anterior dislocation of the mandibular condyle.

Dislocations may be caused by extrinsic forces, such as a punch or kick directed at the mandible, especially when the mouth is open, or intrinsic (self-induced) forces, such as opening the mouth wide on yawning or eating. In these latter cases the predisposing cause is laxity of the capsule and its ligaments, which allows excessive movement. It is well to remember that the TMJ is frequently dislocated while intubating a patient under a general anaesthetic.

The patient with a bilateral dislocation presents with an anterior open bite, but unlike what happens in bilateral fracture dislocations, the mandible protrudes forward, with very limited movement (Fig. 5.20). The patient often experiences pain in the region of the temporal fossae rather than the TMJ region. There is great difficulty in swallowing, and drooling of saliva is common. Dislocation may be treated without sedation or general anaesthetic, depending on the duration of the dislocation.

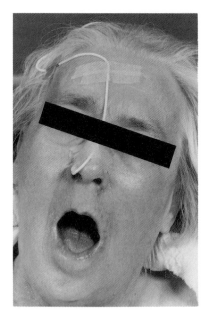

Fig. 5.20 • Anterior open bite as seen in bilateral temporomandibular joint dislocation.

Muscle spasm around the joint can make reduction difficult if considerable time has elapsed. Dislocation of short standing—that is within the first hour or so—can often be treated without any sedation or general anaesthetic, whereas longer-standing dislocation almost invariably requires sedation and muscle-relaxants (in the form of intravenous diazepam) or general anaesthetic for reduction to be successful.

With the patient sitting, or lying down if under general anaesthetic, the operator after explaining the procedure to be attempted positions himself or herself in front of or behind the patient and then presses down the thumbs (covered with gauze for protection) on the occlusal surface of the lower molar teeth or the retromolar region of the mandible on each side, whilst at the same time cupping the chin with the fingers of both hands, elevating the chin, and pushing the mandible posteriorly. This should slip the condyle head back over the eminentia and into the glenoid fossa on each side (Fig. 5.21).

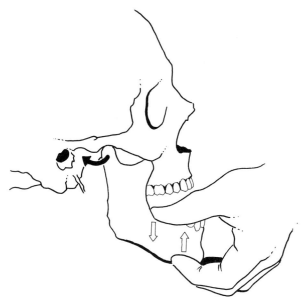

Fig. 5.21 • Reduction of temporomandibular joint dislocation.

Patients should then be advised not to yawn or to open their mouths widely for at least twenty-four hours.

Chronic recurrent dislocations

The condyle may dislocate several times a day, owing to excessive laxity of the capsule. Most of these dislocations are self-reduced by the affected patients; but some require professional help. In confused patients with chronic recurrent dislocation, a barrel elasticated bandage is sometimes helpful in the short term.

In the long term, however, surgery in the form of enlarging the eminentia by osteotomy, or grafting bone to stop the condyle slipping over it, or capsulorrhapy (tightening the capsule) can be of help to some of these patients.

CHAPTER 6

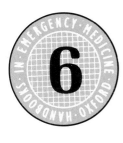

Assessment and treatment of fractures of the middle third of the facial skeleton

Key points in fractures of the middle third of the facial skeleton

1 The middle third of the facial skeleton lies between the frontal bone and the base of the skull above and the mandible below, and comprises the upper jaw, teeth, nose, and maxillary and ethmoidal air sinuses.
2 The majority of middle-third facial fractures result from road-traffic accidents, but they may also be associated with interpersonal assault and sporting injuries.
3 Displaced fractures of the facial skeleton can result in respiratory obstruction, which can be relieved by manual manipulation.
4 Head injuries and cervical-spine injuries may be associated with middle-third fractures, and should always be considered as a possibility.
5 The contents of the superior orbital fissure and the optic nerve may also be injured in fractures of the middle third of the facial skeleton.
6 Prophylactic antibiotics should be used in the treatment of middle-third fractures, especially as compound base-of-skull fractures are commonly associated with this type of injury.
7 Facial deformity, with marked facial bruising and swelling, subconjunctival ecchymosis, and infra-orbital nerve anaesthesia are important clinical features of central middle-third fractures.

Introduction

The number of patients seen in Accident and Emergency Departments with facial trauma is increasing. Injuries of the facial bony skeleton are common, accounting for approximately 35 per cent of all bony injuries. Undergraduate medical teaching on the assessment and management of facial injuries is currently minimal. This is unfortunate, as casualty staff are often required to attend to serious facial injuries, and any doctor may need to administer urgent roadside treatment to a road-traffic accident victim with extensive facial injuries.

Surgical anatomy

The middle third of the facial skeleton lies between the frontal bone and the base of the skull above and the mandible below (Fig. 6.1). It consists of 18 bones—two midline bones (vomer and ethmoid) and eight pairs of bones (maxillae, zygomas, zygomatic processes of the temporal bones, palatine bones, lacrimal bones, nasal bones, pterygoid plates of the sphenoids, and inferior conchae).

The middle third of the face includes the upper jaw and teeth, the nose, and the maxillary and ethmoidal air sinuses. The infra-orbital nerve and naso-lacrimal duct traverse the upper part of this region. Any of these structures may be injured concomitantly with a middle-third fracture. Neighbouring important structures occasionally involved with mid-facial fractures are the eye and orbital muscles and the meninges and base of the brain.

The individual bones of the middle third are generally thin and fragile; however, in articulation with each other they consist basically of a number of vertical bony struts capable of withstanding large loads applied in a direction perpendicular to the base of the skull, such as occur during chewing. However, in contrast to the inherent strength of the

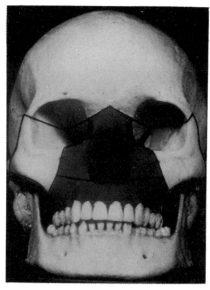

Fig. 6.1 • The middle third of the facial skeleton.

region to withstand forces of mastication applied from below, the middle third of the facial skeleton is relatively weak in a direction parallel to the base of the skull, and is therefore susceptible to injury when forces are applied anteriorly or laterally. Thus on frontal impact the mid-facial skeleton may act as a 'crumple-zone', thereby rendering a form of protection to the cranium and its contents. With severe frontal injury the whole of the mid-facial skeleton can be separated from the base of the skull, and the flail segment is displaced downwards and backwards along the plane of the skull base, producing craniofacial dysjunction.

The muscles attached to the bones of the middle third are mostly muscles of facial expression which insert into facial skin. Therefore in fractures of the middle third (unlike those in mandibular fractures) the muscles do not influence greatly the direction of displacement of the fragments, which is largely due to the direction of the injuring force.

Aetiology of middle-third fractures

The majority of fractures result from road-traffic accidents, personal assaults, sports activities, and accidents at work.

Rowe and Killey (1968) in their study of 629 middle-third injuries found that 296 (47 per cent) resulted from road-traffic accidents, which were the most common single cause of injury. Since the introduction of the seat-belt legislation in 1983, there has been a dramatic shift in the aetiology of injuries. Most maxillofacial surgery units have experienced a decline in the number of middle-third injuries due to road-traffic accidents following the introduction of the seat-belt law. However, the pattern of injuries seen has also changed, with a greater number of more severe middle-third fractures presenting to Accident and Emergency Departments. This shift towards more severe injury is thought to be due to the current survival of vehicle occupants wearing seat-belts who would otherwise not have survived the accident if they had been unrestrained within the motor vehicle. Rapidly re-sponding emergency services and on-scene resuscitation have also contributed to the better survival prospects of multiply-injured patients.

Whilst the number of patients with middle-third injuries due to road-traffic accidents has been reduced, the total number of patients with mid-facial trauma has increased. This alarming statistic is unfortunately the result of a more violent society, with rising numbers of middle-third injuries resulting from assault. Sporting injuries to the face tend to be less serious than those due to assault or road-traffic acci-dents; however, those sports which are more likely to be associated with middle-third fractures are rugby, football, and cricket.

Classification of middle-third fractures

• **Scheme of assessment and management**

A simplified classification:

1. Dento-alveolar fractures.

2. Nasal complex fractures (including naso-ethmoidal injuries).

3. Zygomatic complex fractures (zygoma and associated articulations with the frontal bone, maxilla, and zygomatic process of the temporal bone).

4. Le Fort I (low-level fracture).

5. Le Fort II (pyramidal or infrazygomatic fracture).

6. Le Fort III (high-level, suprazygomatic fracture; craniofacial dysjunction).

Le Fort, a Parisian Surgeon, produced his classification of middle-third injuries in 1901 by dropping cadavers on to their faces and examining the resulting fracture lines (Fig. 6.2).

Whilst his classification is extremely useful and is in widespread use today, it should be remembered that classical fractures occur infrequently, and bilateral fractures are seldom symmetrical. Also, there is virtually never a single fracture segment. The more typical pattern of a severe middle-third injury is a displaced comminuted fracture with sixty or seventy separate bony fragments.

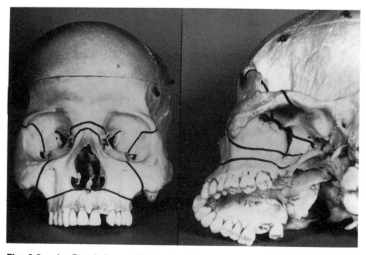

Fig. 6.2 • Le Fort I, II, and III fracture-lines.

Whilst the maxillary teeth and surrounding alveolar bone and the zygomas (malars) do form part of the middle third of the facial skeleton, a fracture of these areas in isolation is, rather confusingly, not usually referred to as 'a middle-third fracture' in the clinical setting. This term is usually reserved for the Le Fort I, II, and III fractures and naso-ethmoidal injuries.

The remainder of this chapter will deal with the assessment and management of patients with middle-third fractures, except for fractures of the zygomatic complex, which are covered in Chapter 7.

Scheme of assessment and management of middle-third facial fractures

1. Initial rapid assessment
2. Resuscitation and primary care
3. Definitive history and examination
4. Radiological imaging
5. Initial treatment
6. Definitive treatment of fractures

The general assessment and resuscitation of traumatised patients is dealt with in Chapter 4, and therefore the following is restricted to the management of the middle-third injury alone.

History and extraoral examination

- ### Facial examination

A full history should be taken whenever possible, including the past medical history, known allergies, and current medication.

The nature of the injury force should be established where possible, as this may give an indication as to the severity of the injuries likely to have been sustained.

Facial examination

Inspection

The face should be examined from the front, the side, and also from above, by standing behind the patient. The typical appearance of a severe middle-third fracture is a flattened elongated face (dish-face) due to the displacement of the mid-facial skeleton downwards and backwards along the cranial base (Fig. 6.3). Shortly afterwards facial oedema will rapidly accumulate, causing the lax soft tissues of the face to swell alarmingly, giving the whole face a rounded appearance, aptly described as ballooning (Fig. 6.4). Later, bilateral circumorbital bruising develops, producing the so-called 'panda facies' or 'racoon-sign', typical of a severe middle-third fracture (Fig. 6.5).

The face should be inspected from the front and from above for asymmetry—for instance an area of flattening over a cheek-bone (zygoma) due to a fracture of the zygomatic

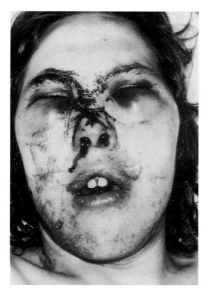

Fig. 6.3 • An elongated face with marked periorbital swelling and CSF rhinorrhoea.

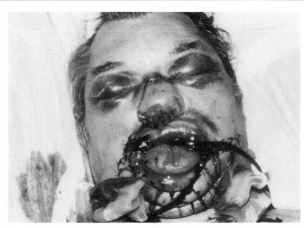

Fig. 6.4 • Ballooning of the face associated with a severe middle-third injury.

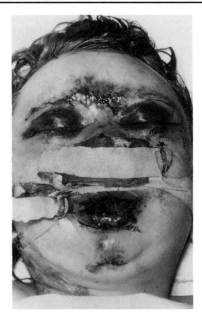

Fig. 6.5 • Periorbital bruising producing the 'panda facies' or 'racoon sign'.

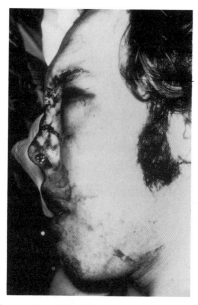

Fig. 6.6 • Dish-face and saddle-bridge nose deformity.

complex or a Le Fort III fracture. A deviated nose due to an isolated nasal complex fracture may be obvious when viewed from above. The nasal bridge may be severely depressed as a result of a frontal injury, producing the saddle-bridge nose deformity of a naso-ethmoidal injury (Fig. 6.6). Epistaxis usually occurs with any middle-third fracture. Naso-ethmoidal and Le Fort II and III fractures may involve the floor of the anterior cranial fossa in the region of the cribriform plate of the ethmoid bone. Adjacent structures which may be traumatized are the olfactory nerves, giving rise to anosmia (loss of sense of smell), and the meninges, whereby a tear in the dural layer can give rise to a cerebrospinal fluid (CSF) leak. Pure CSF is clear, but by the time it reaches the face through the nostrils (CSF rhinorrhoea) it is usually straw-coloured. The CSF does not clot, and may drip persistently from the nose or ooze on to the upper lip, producing 'tramlining'—the blood on the upper lip is pushed aside by the CSF, which runs down between the two red tramlines. CSF can reliably be differentiated from a serous or mucous discharge by a positive reaction for glucose on stick testing. Alternatively, the CSF may track backwards to the nasopharynx, where it is difficult to recognize, though the patient may complain of a salty taste. It is important to recognize a CSF leak because of the potential risk of meningitis, and therefore in such cases prophylactic chemotherapy against this potential infection is indicated. With a severe mid-facial injury a CSF leak should be assumed and appropriate prophylaxis should be commenced (see p. 117).

Careful ophthalmological examination is mandatory. The pupillary level is assessed from the front with the patient's head in the 'neutral' position. Alteration in pupillary level could indicate a fracture of the orbital floor. The eyes are examined for any obvious penetrating injuries and for the presence of subconjuctival haemorrhage, which is bright red and can vary in degree from a flame-shaped area to total coverage of the visible sclera. A fracture involving one of the orbital walls produces subconjuctival haemorrhage which has no posterior limit, whereas the subconjunctival haemorrhage associated with a 'black eye' or contused globe does have a posterior limit.

The eyes should be examined for:

1. Visual acuity.
2. Range of movements and diplopia (III, IV, or VI cranial nerve lesions, extraocular muscle-trapping).
3. Pupillary size, symmetry, and direct/consensual light reflex (II and III nerve lesions).
4. Fundoscopically, for papilloedema, vitreous haemorrhages, hyphaema, retinal tears, and optic nerve-head ischaemia.

The distance between the medial canthus of the eyes should be measured as an indicator of a **traumatic telecanthus**—a severe frontal injury such as occurs with a naso-ethmoidal fracture can disrupt the normal attachment of the medial canthal ligament (part of the suspensory ligament of the globe) from the medial wall of the orbit. The detached ligament, and usually a portion of bone to which it is attached, is retracted laterally. The distance between the medial canthi of the eyes (intercanthal distance) is normally equal to the width of one palpebral fissure (between 3.3 and 3.5 cm). This distance is increased when a traumatic telecanthal injury is present (Fig. 6.7). It is important to recognize this injury, as failure to correct it surgically results in significant deformity.

Palpation

This is performed bimanually and symmetrically, which enables direct comparison of both sides of the face. It is best to stand in front of the patient and gently palpate the bony margins and prominences for areas of tenderness, step deformity, movement, or crepitus. It is usual to commence with the superior orbital margins, and then the lateral and inferior margins, followed by the nasal bones, the zygomas, the zygomatic arches, and the remainder of the facial skeleton.

If deep facial lacerations are present it may be possible to palpate gently beneath the laceration with a gloved finger to detect an underlying fracture of the antero-lateral surface of

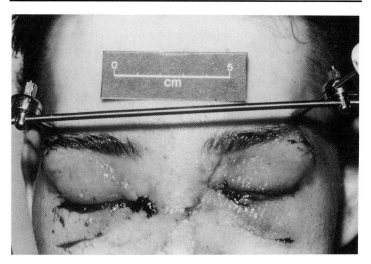

Fig. 6.7 • Traumatic telecanthus.

the maxilla, infra-orbital margin, or fronto-zygomatic region.

The characteristic crepitus of surgical emphysema may be palpable within the soft tissues of the face, especially in the infra-orbital region; this indicates an underlying fracture communicating with an air sinus.

If a Le Fort II or III fracture is suspected then abnormal movement at the naso-frontal junction can usually be detected by gently rocking the maxilla in an antero-posterior direction with the index finger and thumb of the right hand firmly holding the upper incisor teeth (Fig. 6.8). Similarly, movement at the fronto-zygomatic junction may be palpable with the same manœuvre in the presence of a Le Fort III fracture (Fig. 6.9).

Le Fort II and III and high Le Fort I fractures often traumatize the infra-orbital nerve in its canal or at the foramen, producing a facial paraesthesia, or less commonly anaesthesia over the cheek. Any sensory loss is detected by loss of light touch sensation to cotton wool and pin-prick sensation to a blunted needle.

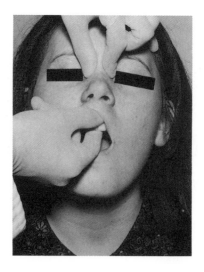

Fig. 6.8 • Examining for movement in the fronto-nasal suture region.

Intraoral examination

- Inspection   Palpation   Percussion

The oral cavity should be carefully examined with a good light source.

Inspection

By asking the patient to bite together gently the occlusion (or bite) should be examined for posterior gagging. This is a premature contact of the posterior teeth on closing, so that the anterior teeth do not meet—anterior open bite. This is due to the displacement and rotation of the fractured maxilla. Posterior gagging of the occlusion is not exclusive to maxillary fractures, as the same appearance can result from bilateral mandibular condylar fractures.

The oral mucosa should be inspected for lacerations or areas of bruising which may indicate an underlying fracture, as in the following examples:

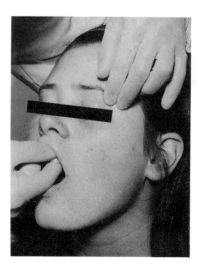

Fig. 6.9 • Examining for movement at the fronto-zygomatic suture.

- Laceration or haematoma over the midline of the hard palate may indicate a split palate.
- Bruising over the greater palatine foramen associated with a fracture of the pterygoid plates.
- Bruising over the base of the zygomatic buttress (in the upper buccal sulcus) indicating a fracture of the zygoma.

The upper teeth should be inspected for a step deformity, which can occur with a split palate or an isolated fracture of the tooth-bearing portion of the maxilla (dento-alveolar fracture). A note is made of the teeth present and teeth missing, and of any fractured or mobile teeth.

Palpation

The upper teeth and alveolus should be gently grasped and rocked to elicit abnormal movement of the maxilla or alveolus. It is sufficient to perform this once in the midline and once on each side towards the back teeth. At the same time it may be possible to demonstrate a split palate.

A fingertip (usually the index finger's) should be passed over the oral mucosa that is applied to the maxilla, by running the finger along the buccal sulcus between the cheek and the upper teeth to permit the detection of tenderness, step deformity, and abnormal mobility.

Percussion

Tapping the upper teeth with a hard instrument such as the end of a dental mirror is said to produce a 'cracked-cup' note in the presence of a maxillary fracture. However, the value of this test is limited, and it can be painful for the patient; and therefore percussion of the maxillary teeth is not recommended.

Summary of clinical features which may be present

(A) *Isolated nasal fracture*

1. Flattened or deviated nose

2. Swelling
3. Epistaxis
4. Septal deviation
5. Septal haematoma
6. Mouthbreathing (obstructed nasal airway)
7. Tenderness over nasal bones
8. Mobility

(B) *Naso-ethmoidal fracture*

1. Flattened nasal bridge with splaying of nasal complex
2. Saddle-shaped deformity of nose from side
3. Traumatic telecanthus
4. Circumorbital oedema and ecchymosis (initially more marked medially)
5. Subconjunctival haemorrhage (especially medially)
6. Epistaxis
7. CSF rhinorrhoea
8. Possible supra-orbital/supratrochlear nerve paraesthesia
9. Tenderness, crepitus, and mobility of nasal complex
10. Overlying laceration

(C) *Dento-alveolar fracture*

1. Stepped alignment of teeth
2. Derangement of occlusion
3. Lacerations of gingiva/mucosa
4. Overlying bruising/haematoma of mucosa
5. Mobile segment of teeth
6. Palpable fracture in buccal sulcus
7. Oedematous lips
8. Ragged laceration of inner aspect of lips and cheek

(D) *Le Fort I fracture*

1. Lengthening of face (due to dropped maxillary segment)
2. Bruising within buccal sulcus

3. Asymmetry of tooth alignment when viewed from the front (one side dropped lower than the other)
4. Derangement of occlusion and shift in upper midline
5. Mobile maxillary fragment involving the whole of the tooth-bearing area, with tenderness and crepitus
6. Lacerations of the upper lip or oral mucosa
7. ± Split palate

(E) *Le Fort II fracture*
1. Gross facial oedema (ballooning)
2. Elongated face with flattening
3. Circumorbital oedema and ecchymosis
4. Subconjuctival haemorrhage (medially)
5. Diplopia
6. Epistaxis
7. CSF rhinorrhoea
8. Surgical emphysema
9. Gagging of the occlusion posteriorly
10. Anterior open bite
11. Infra-orbital nerve sensory loss
12. Mobility of central 'pyramidal' area of face on bimanual testing
13. Palpable fracture 'step' of infra-orbital margin
14. ± Nasal complex fracture
15. ± Split palate
16. Occasionally conjunctival chemosis, enophthalmos, or limitation of eye movement

(F) *Le Fort III fractures*

A Le Fort II and Le Fort III fracture can appear similar on initial examination, but the latter is obviously a more severe injury, and also involves the lateral region of the middle third.

Therefore the following clinical features should be added to those in (E) above:

17. Flattening over zygomatic bones
18. Mobility and tenderness of zygomas
19. Steep deformity of the fronto-zygomatic sutures and over the zygomatic arch, with tenderness
20. Palpable movement of the zygoma at the fronto-zygomatic suture on rocking the maxilla
21. Alteration in pupillary level and 'hooding of the globe of the eye' as the upper lid droops down with an inferiorly displaced globe.

It should be noted that patients with any of the Le Fort fractures may complain of an inability to open the mouth. The reason for this is that the mandible is actually already in the 'open' position, owing to the fractured maxilla's being driven down on to it, giving rise to the elongated facial appearance. If the maxillary fragment is gently manipulated upwards and forwards back into its anatomical position then the mouth-open position becomes obvious, and the patient is then able to close the mouth.

Radiological imaging

• **Interpretation of facial radiographs   Computed tomography**

As was mentioned previously, if a cervical spine injury is suspected then radiographs of the whole of the cervical spine must take priority over facial views.

Interpretation of facial radiographs

The interpretation of facial radiographs is often difficult for a number of reasons:

(1) complex skeletal anatomy;
(2) superimposition of bones;
(3) masking of fracture lines by soft-tissue oedema and maxillary sinuses filled with blood;
(4) a restless, agitated, or confused patient, resulting in poor-quality films; and

(5) a possible limitation of views as a result of cervical spine injury.

The minimal radiographs required are:

(1) the lateral skull and the facial bones; and

(2) a 15° occipitomental view,

plus the following views, which provide a full radiographic assessment:

(3) 30° occipitomental;

(4) postero-anterior facial bones;

(5) submento-vertex;

(6) nasal bones; and

(7) intraoral.

It is unwise to place too much emphasis on the diagnostic sensitivity of facial radiographs for fractures. Careful interpretation of the films should enable confirmation of a provisional diagnosis based on good clinical examination techniques.

The single most useful film for viewing a middle-third fracture is the occipitomental (Fig. 6.10). It is important to compare each side with the other, and with this in mind it is helpful to follow the 'four curvilinear lines' of McGregor and Campbell (Fig. 6.11).

The *first line* passes from one fronto-zygomatic (FZ) suture across the top of the orbits to the opposite FZ suture. Look for separation at the FZ suture or a break in the normal smooth contour of the superior orbital margin.

The *second line* runs along the zygomatic arch across the inferior border of the orbit (above the maxillary air sinus), across the nose to the opposite inferior orbital margin and zygomatic arch. Again attention is focused on the cortical surface of the bones for a break in continuity or a step defect. The zygomatic arch and inferior orbital margin are common sites of fracture in middle-third injuries.

The *third line* begins from the head of one mandibular condyle and crosses the tip of the coronoid process to the lateral wall of the maxillary air sinus, passes through the

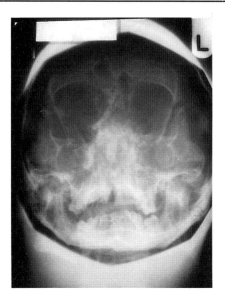

Fig. 6.10 • Radiograph (15° occipitomental view) demonstrating a Le Fort III fracture.

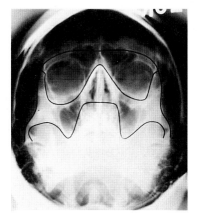

Fig. 6.11 • Systematic inspection of an occipitomental view.

sinus to the floor of the nasal cavity, and follows the same course on the opposite side. Look for fractures of the lateral wall of the sinus (Le Fort I, II, or III fractures) and for opacification of the sinus, indicating the presence of blood. The 'hanging-drop' sign of an orbital floor blow-out fracture due to herniation of the orbital contents into the air sinus may be recognized.

The *fourth line* runs along the curved junction of the upper and lower teeth, and may reveal a step in the normally smooth contour line if a dento-alveolar fracture or split palate is present.

The lateral film of the facial bones is inspected for fracture of the bony struts which run from the upper teeth region to the base of the skull. Look specifically for fractures of the anterior and posterior walls of the air sinuses (maxillary and frontal) and for fractures of the pterygoid plates behind the maxilla (Fig. 6.12). The middle third of the face may be pushed back, with posterior gagging of the occlusion and an anterior open bite seen on the lateral film (Fig. 6.13). The nasal complex should be inspected for sites of fracture.

Computed tomography (CT)

Accurate assessment of middle-third facial fractures has greatly improved with the introduction of CT scans. This has helped enormously with the planning of definitive surgery, and allows the most appropriate surgical approach and methods of immobilization of the fractures to be decided well in advance. CT scans have a number of advantages over plain radiographs and tomograms:

1. No need for difficult positioning of the patient.

2. No movement of the cervical spine.

3. Does not compromise continuing ventilatory measures.

4. High-quality images unaffected by soft-tissue oedema and haemorrhage.

5. Better definition of 'difficult' areas, such as the naso-ethmoidal region and the orbital floor (Fig. 6.14).

6. Concurrent injuries, such as intracranial or cervical-spine injuries, can be evaluated at the same time.

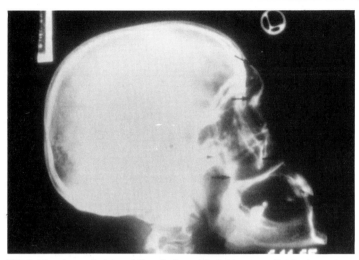

Fig. 6.12 • Lateral view of the skull and facial bones, demonstrating sites of fracture.

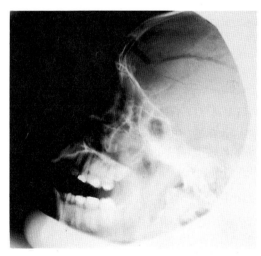

Fig. 6.13 • Central middle-third fracture with displacement. Note posterior gagging and anterior open bite. Linear skull fracture is also evident.

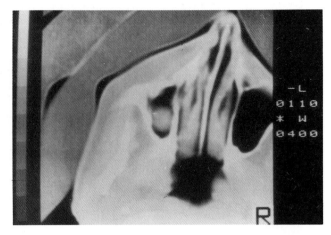

Fig. 6.14 • CT scan (transverse slice). Note orbital floor blow-out, with orbital contents within left maxillary antrum.

It is possible with many scanners to produce three-dimensional images of the facial skeleton which can be of value when planning surgery. For assessment of middle-third fractures 3-D reconstructions are of little benefit over plain CT scans.

Initial treatment

- **Avoid nose-blowing   Prophylaxis of infection   Pain relief   Facial lacerations   Referral and transfer to a maxillofacial unit**

Avoid nose-blowing

Blowing the nose in the presence of a middle-third fracture which communicates with an air sinus or the nasal cavity can produce sudden dramatic surgical emphysema of the soft tissues of the face. There is also the potential danger of driving microorganisms into the fracture site or soft tissues, or intracranially through a basal skull fracture.

Prophylaxis of infection

Most middle-third fractures communicate with an air sinus, the nose, or the mouth, or externally through a laceration, and are therefore compound fractures. Prevention of infection within such contaminated fractures is therefore warranted. Parenteral penicillin (benzylpencillin), if not contraindicated, is a good first choice.

If a cerebro-spinal fluid leak is suspected then chemo-prophylaxis against meningitis is necessary. A sulphonamide such as sulphadimidine is administered parenterally, in combination with a penicillin.

All patients must have their tetanus immunization checked, and if no booster has been given within the last 10 years then a tetanus-toxoid booster is administered.

Pain relief

Patients with extensive middle-third fractures do not usually complain of severe pain. If pain is a significant feature, how-ever, then it is usually due to mobility of the fracture, and the best pain relief is obtained by temporary immobilization of the fracture with dental wiring or by infiltration around the fracture site with a local anaesthetic. If systemic anal-gesia is required then narcotic agents such as morphine or pethidine should be avoided because of the possibility of masking early symptoms and signs of raised intracranial pressure. Diclofenac sodium (Voltarol) is a suitable alterna-tive, given intramuscularly.

Facial lacerations

These should be cleaned with saline or antiseptic solution and covered with a dry absorbent dressing. No facial soft tissue should ever be excised, no matter how compromised the vascular supply may appear. Skin lacerations should not be initially sutured, as they may allow palpation of a fracture beneath the wound edges, and will also require thorough de-bridement, often under general anaesthesia. A laceration may also be useful to allow access to a fracture site for open reduc-tion and direct fixation—especially lacerations of the lips and cheeks, which can provide excellent access to a fracture.

Referral and transfer to a maxillofacial unit

All patients with a Le Fort I, II, or III fracture, a naso-ethmoidal fracture, or a significant dento-alveolar fracture should be admitted immediately to hospital following referral to a maxillofacial surgeon. Uncomplicated nasal bone fractures without septal haematoma can be allowed home, with arrangements for review in the maxillofacial surgery department.

If a maxillofacial department is not present in the referring hospital then transfer is necessary to the appropriate hospital. The patient must be fully assessed and actively resuscitated and stabilized prior to transfer. Immediate transfer during the night is mostly unnecessary and often undesirable, and can safely await daylight hours so long as the patient is carefully monitored. All inter-hospital transfers should be by ambulance with accompanying medical personnel. All clinical notes and radiographs should accompany the patient. The referring doctor must communicate directly with the receiving maxillofacial surgeon before transfer.

Definitive treatment

• **Timing of surgery   Nasal fractures   Naso-ethmoidal fractures   Dento-alveolar fractures**

The principles of treatment are no different to those applied to any fracture, namely:

• reduction;
• immobilization; and
• rehabilitation.

A period of immobilization of around four weeks is usually sufficient to allow good bony union. Non-union due to infection is extremely uncommon, because of the excellent blood-supply of the mid-face.

The majority of patients with a cerebro-spinal fluid leak complicating a middle-third fracture will not require formal exploration and repair of the dural tear. Most leaks will stop after satisfactory definitive treatment of the fracture. If the leak continues after the seventh postoperative day then a neurosurgical opinion should be sought.

Timing of surgery

The majority of patients do not require immediate surgery, and indeed delaying definitive treatment for 2–5 days can be beneficial in that it allows the general condition of the patient to be observed and stabilized, further specific or repeat radiographs to be obtained, facial oedema to subside, and time for consultation with an anaesthetist familiar with head and neck surgery.

Any facial lacerations, however, should be closed within 24 hours of injury, as beyond this period the incidence of wound infection rises dramatically.

If the patient is taken to theatre for a concurrent injury such as limb fractures or emergency laparotomy, then the maxillofacial surgeon should be informed so that primary treatment of the facial fracture may be undertaken at the same time. Impressions of the teeth may be taken to enable construction of accurately fitting splints, and facial lacerations can be formally repaired. Temporary or even definitive immobilization of the facial fracture may be performed.

Nasal fractures

Again it is usually wise to review the patient after 48–72 hours in order to allow initial oedema to subside. If a septal haematoma is present, however, then this requires immediate evacuation to avoid subsequent necrosis and collapse of the septal cartilage. Any previous history of nasal trauma should be ascertained and enquiry should be made as to the previous shape of the nose (a photograph is useful in this respect). A deviated nose may be the result of a previous 'old' injury, and attempted reduction will then be unsuccessful.

Displaced nasal cartilages can often be relocated by digital manipulation. Fractures of the nasal bones and frontal processes of the maxillae, which are often associated with a buckled or fractured nasal septum, should be reduced by closed manipulation with Walsham's nasal forceps and

Asche's septal forceps under general anaesthesia. Haemostasis is achieved with intranasal packing of 2.5 cm ribbon gauze impregnated with Whitehead's varnish or bismuth iodoform and paraffin paste (BIPP). External splintage is often required, and the T-shaped plaster-of-paris splint is in common use. The nasal packing is removed after 24 hours and the external splint after 10 days, by which time it is usually a poor fit as a result of reduced oedema. Premade thermoplastic splints are ill-fitting and unsuitable for adequate stabilization.

If other fractures of the mid-face are present then these should be dealt with initially before attempting manipulation of the nasal fracture.

Naso-ethmoidal fractures

Less severe naso-ethmoidal fractures can be missed and incorrectly diagnosed as an isolated nasal fracture. A high index of suspicion is necessary in order not to miss this serious injury. Depressed fractures of the frontal bone, severe nasal deformity (especially saddle nose), traumatic telecanthus or CSF rhinorrhoea should alert the examining surgeon to the possibility of a naso-ethmoidal injury. With definite naso-ethmoidal fractures, a CSF leak should be assumed to be present even if it is not clinically demonstrable, and appropriate chemoprophylaxis should be commenced. An intercanthal distance of greater than 35 mm is suggestive of traumatic telecanthus, and measurements approaching 40 mm are almost diagnostic.

Closed manipulation of these injuries gives a poor result, with a high incidence of persistent telecanthus and residual nasal deformity postoperatively. The results of secondary surgery of these abnormalities are also disappointing. Therefore early open reduction of naso-ethmoidal injuries is generally advocated. The naso-ethmoidal region can be exposed through an existing laceration, which may require extension, or through a surgical incision such as a mid-line vertical, H-shaped, or W-shaped incision. If the naso-ethmoidal fracture is associated with fractures of the frontal bone or if access to the superior, medial, or lateral orbital walls is required, then the bicoronal flap (Fig. 6.15) would be indicated. This useful

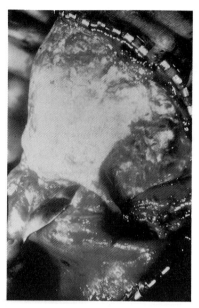

Fig. 6.15 • Bicoronal flap, with exposure of frontal bone and orbital roofs.

flap provides excellent exposure of this region, and allows relatively good access to the orbital walls.

Following exposure of the injury, it is usual to find extensive comminution of the naso-ethmoidal region, although the nasal bridge may be intact, and consequently driven into the ethmoidal region between the orbits (Fig. 6.16). The nasal bridge is elevated back into position and stabilized by direct wiring, or occasionally by mini-plates to the frontal bone (Fig. 6.17). The remaining multiple fragments are then reduced individually, aligned, and directly wired both to each other and to the surrounding intact bony skeleton. It is unusual for there to be any missing fragments of bone.

The medial canthal ligaments must be formally identified. If a canthal ligament is detached from its bony insertion upon the frontal process of the maxilla, then it must be repositioned and stabilized in the correct anatomical position

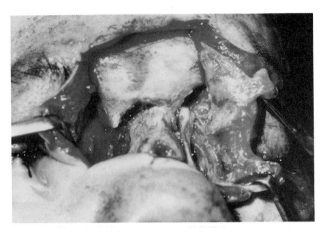

Fig. 6.16 naso-ethmoidal fracture at operation.

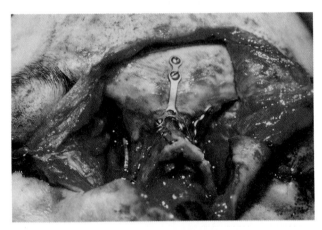

Fig. 6.17 • Fracture reduced and stabilized with mini-plate.

by wiring the canthal ligament to the opposite anterior lacrimal crest—transnasal canthopexy. If both canthal ligaments are detached then the telecanthus is corrected by means of wiring the two medial canthal ligaments to each other, again transnasally.

Dento-alveolar fractures

These injuries involve the teeth and their supporting bone— the alveolus. The fractured segment may be completely avulsed, or more usually is retained, and remains viable because of an attached mucoperiosteal vascular pedicle. Such fragments are well worth repositioning into the correct occlusal relationship, often under local anaesthesia, and are then immobilized with an acrylic splint which accurately fits the upper teeth. Alternative methods of immobilization are metal arch bars which are wired to the teeth, including the fracture segment, and cast silver splints which can be cemented or wired directly to the alveolar bone.

The fragment is immobilized for 4–6 weeks, after which time the dento-alveolar fracture has usually firmly united.

Maxillary fractures (Le Fort I, II, and III)

• Methods of fixation

Pre-operative planning is essential for all mid-face fractures. The operation should therefore proceed as a series of planned stages, and the likely methods of fixation to be used should have been decided in advance. When extensive facial reconstruction is anticipated then elective tracheostomy may be performed initially.

Subsequent treatment of the facial injuries proceeds according to the following sequence:

1. Reduce and stabilize the mandible.
2. Disimpact any concomitant fracture of the zygomatic complex.
3. Disimpact and reduce the fractured maxilla.
4. Immobilize the reduced maxilla in the correct occlusal relationship to the mandible.
5. Immobilize the zygomatic fractures.
6. Reconstruct the orbital walls and the naso-ethmoidal region.
7. Soft-tissue repair.

The maxilla is disimpacted and reduced with Rowe's maxillary disimpaction forceps (Fig. 6.18). These consist of a pair of cranked forceps, each with a large padded blade, which is positioned intraorally against the roof of the mouth, and a smaller non-padded blade, which is passed along the nasal floor. With the operator standing behind the patient's head, both forceps are firmly grasped, and, while an assistant supports the patient's head, the maxilla is disimpacted and advanced in an antero-superior direction to achieve the correct anatomical relationship. Considerable force is often required to disimpact a Le Fort II or III fracture.

The reduced maxilla is immobilized by means of external fixation or internal fixation, or by application of both methods. Over the last decade there has been a change in emphasis, with a shift away from external fixation methods towards rigid internal fixation.

Methods of fixation of maxillary fractures

External fixation
Craniomaxillary—Royal Berkshire halo frame (Figs 6.19 and 6.20)
—Levant frame (Fig. 6.21)

Craniomandibular—Mount Vernon box frame (Fig. 6.22)

Internal fixation
Direct transosseous wiring

Suspension wires—circumzygomatic
—frontomandibular
—infra-orbital
—central frontal
Transfixation Kirschner wires
Bone-plate osteosynthesis

External fixation
This is achieved by immobilizing the middle-third fracture between adjacent stable bones of the skull. Craniomaxillary fixation is a means of rigidly suspending the maxilla from the skull vault by connecting rods which are secured to either a halo-type frame or a Levant frame. The halo frame is attached to the skull by four diametrically opposed screw

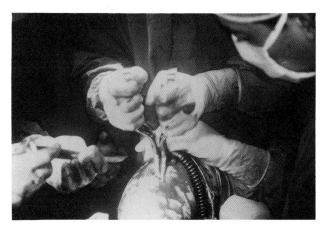

Fig. 6.18 • Maxillary disimpaction.

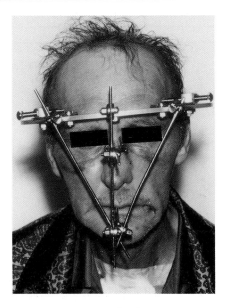

Fig. 6.19 • Craniomaxillary external fixation.

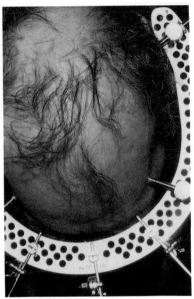

Fig. 6.20 • Royal Berkshire halo frame.

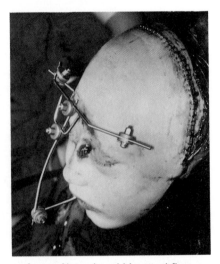

Fig. 6.21 • Levant frame. Note closed bicoronal flap.

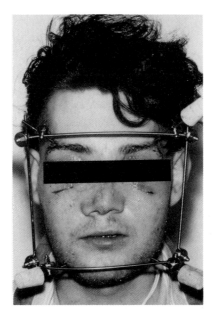

Fig. 6.22 • Craniomandibular box frame.

pins which penetrate the scalp to engage the outer cortical surface of the cranium, whilst the Levant frame is secured by two self-tapping pins inserted through the outer cortex into the cancellous bone of the external angular process of the frontal bone. The connecting rods are rigidly attached to an anteriorly projecting metal bar which is itself connected to an arch bar wired to the upper teeth, a cast silver splint fitting over the upper teeth; or, if the patient is edentulous, the bar can be connected to a modified upper denture which is wired to the maxilla.

Craniomandibular fixation is a rigid connection of the mandible to the cranium with four extra oral pins—two inserted above the maxillary fracture into the external angular processes of the frontal bone, and two below the maxilla into a stable mandible. The pins are rigidly connected, so that the fractured maxilla is 'sandwiched' between the skull vault and the mandible by this box frame.

External fixation methods are not sufficiently rigid to be used by themselves, and further stability has to be achieved by locking the jaws together (intermaxillary fixation) with interdental eyelet wiring.

Internal fixation

Transosseous wiring is frequently used as a method of internal fixation; however, it also provides insufficient rigidity by itself, and is therefore used in conjunction with other methods of fixation, such as internal skeletal suspension or external skeletal fixation. Suitable sites for the placement of transosseous wires are:

(1) the fronto-zygomatic suture;

(2) the fronto-nasal suture;

(3) the fronto-maxillary suture; and

(4) the infra-orbital margin.

Internal fixation by suspension wiring is achieved by suspending the fractured maxilla with stainless steel wires from a stable part of the facial skeleton, such as the zygomatic arches, the external angular processes of the frontal bone, or the infra-orbital margin, or from a single screw which is inserted in the middle of the frontal bone, just above the frontal sinus. A common disadvantage of all the techniques of internal suspension is that the stabilizing force acts in an upwards and backwards direction, which may encourage early relapse of the reduced maxilla. Intermaxillary fixation is therefore necessary in order to reduce the risk of fracture relapse.

Facial transfixation with Kirschner wires is generally not an acceptable method of fixation because of the poor degree of control of the fragments. It is however, a rapid and relatively simple technique that requires little equipment. The technique may have value in the treatment of maxillary fractures in medically unfit or elderly patients, where a short anaesthetic time would be advantageous. The Le Fort II fracture is most suitable for transfixation, whilst the technique is of no value in the treatment of a Le Fort I fracture. The K-wire is driven through the stable zygoma on one side, through the reduced maxilla, and into the stable zygoma on the other side, thus forming a 'kebab' immobilization of the maxilla. The degree of stability and control of the fracture can be improved by inserting a second K-wire at a different angle, producing a criss-cross pattern of the K-wires.

The last two decades have seen major developments in the management of facial fractures, following the introduction of bone-plate osteosynthesis. The use of bone plates was initially directed at the mandible, to enable rigid fixation of mandibular fractures. The introduction of mini-plate systems has allowed these same techniques of osteosynthesis to be applied to middle-third fractures of the facial skeleton (Fig. 6.23). Fracture fixation with mini-plates produces rigid stable internal fixation, and additional fixation is often unnecessary. Whilst it is usual for the occlusion to be stabilized initially with intermaxillary fixation this can usually be removed after the first few postoperative days, thereby allowing the patient to open the mouth. This is of obvious advantage to the patient, allowing normal dietary intake,

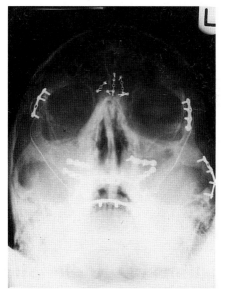

Fig. 6.23 • Internal fixation of middle-third fractures with mini-plates.

unimpeded speech, and normal oral hygiene measures, and therefore improved comfort for the patient.

The fronto-zygomatic suture is a particularly suitable site for the insertion of a mini-plate, thereby producing a stable platform for the immobilization of Le Fort II and III fractures. The zygomatico-maxillary suture is also a favoured fracture site for plating, and often the bone plate can be inserted through an intraoral incision, which avoids a facial scar.

Thus the current trend is towards the more widespread use of mini-plate systems for the fixation of mid-facial fractures.

Rehabilitation

Maxillofacial rehabilitation should proceed in conjunction with the general rehabilitation of the multiply-injured patient.

The oro-facial rehabilitation of the patient may include:

1. **Restoration of the occlusion**
   (a) New or replacement dentures
   (b) Crowns or bridgework
   (c) Implant systems

2. **Retraining of masticatory muscles**
   (a) Physiotherapy
   (b) Occlusal splints
   (c) Temporomandibular joint surgery

3. **Secondary correction of deformity**
   (a) Scar revision
   (b) Rhinoplasty
   (c) Facial onlay grafts
   (d) Osteotomies
   (e) Prosthetic replacement of eyes, nose, and ears

Complications of middle-third fractures

Non-union of mid-facial fractures is virtually unknown. Complications of severe middle-third fractures are, however, not uncommon, and in a series of 100 patients Bramley (1972) reported the following incidence of complications:

1. Facial scarring (30 per cent)
2. Post-concussional syndrome (24 per cent)
3. Trigeminal nerve sensory defects (24 per cent)
4. Residual cosmetic defect (21 per cent)
5. Anosmia (12 per cent)
6. Epiphora (10 per cent)
7. Persistent diplopia (8 per cent)
8. Loss of eye (7 per cent)
9. Facial nerve palsy (3 per cent)
10. Deafness (1 per cent)

An increasing number of patients with severe mid-facial injuries are presenting to Accident and Emergency Departments. Improved imaging techniques, more cosmetically acceptable surgical approaches, and better methods of fracture fixation, in particular rigid internal fixation, have combined to improve dramatically the management of these patients.

Further reading

Bramley, P. (1972). Long term effects of facial injuries. *Proceedings of the Royal Society of Medicine*, **65(10)**, 916–81.

Rowe, N. L. and Killey, M. C. (1968). *Fractures of the facial skeleton*. Churchill Livingstone, Edinburgh.

CHAPTER 7

Assessment of malar fractures and orbital complications of facial trauma

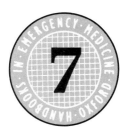

Key points in malar orbital trauma

1 The malar bone and the orbit form the lateral third of the mid-facial skeleton.

2 Malar fractures are the most common type of fracture of the facial skeleton sustained in the British Isles.

3 The globe, optic nerves, the contents of the superior orbital fissure, and the lacrimal apparatus are important anatomical structures which can be involved in malar orbital trauma.

4 The majority of these fractures are caused by interpersonal assault.

5 Remember to examine the eye whenever you see a malar orbital injury.

6 CT scan and MR imaging may help in the diagnosis; but radiographic evaluation is only secondary to systematic clinical examination.

7 Subconjunctival ecchymosis and infra-orbital anaesthesia are two important clinical features of malar orbital injury.

8 The important postoperative care involves nursing upright, regular eye observation, and avoidance of nose-blowing.

9 Retrobulbar haemorrhage should be dealt with immediately.

Surgical anatomy

The malar (the zygomatic bone) and the orbit form the lateral third of the midfacial skeleton. The malar forms the prominence of the cheek, and contributes to the formation of the lateral wall and floor of the orbit. It is quadrangular in shape, with two processes, namely the zygomatico-frontal process superiorly and zygomatico-temporal process laterally. The medial and inferior articulations are to the maxillary bone. Two important sensory nerves, the zygomatico-facial and the zygomatico-temporal, emerge through the lateral and temporal surfaces respectively (Fig. 7.1). The temporalis fascia splits into two sheets approximately 2 cm above the

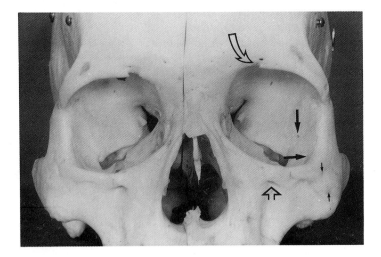

Fig. 7.1 • Osteology of the malar orbital region. On the lateral surface the zygomatico-facial foramina (small arrows) for the passage of the zygomatico-facial nerve and vessels are seen. The orbital surface presents the orifices (large arrows) termed the zygomatico-orbital foramina, one of which leads to the zygomatico-facial and the other to the zygomatico-temporal foramen. Note also the infra-orbital foramen for the passage of the infra-orbital nerve (triangle) and the supra-orbital notch (open arrow) for the passage of the supra-orbital nerve and vessels.

zygomatic arch, and then attaches on either side of the zygomatic arch. The temporal extension of the buccal fat pad fills the gap between these fascial components and the zygomatic arch. This anatomical arrangement is very helpful in the treatment of malar fractures, and also aids the stability of the malar arch.

The orbit is a conical-shaped cavity formed of seven bones. It has four walls and four rims. The orbit contains the globe, the ocular muscles, nerves, vessels, and ligaments. The roof of the orbit separates from the floor of the anterior cranial fossa; the floor forms the roof of the maxillary antrum; and the medial wall lines the ethmoidal air-cells. The lateral wall approximates the temporal fossa, which contains the temporalis muscle. Two types of orbital fractures, described as 'blow-out' and 'blow-in' fractures involve the walls. In the former one or more walls are pushed out, thus increasing the orbital volume. This results in enophthalmos. In the blow-in fracture one or more walls are pushed in, and thus reduce the orbital volume. This may cause proptosis or traumatic exophthalmos.

Several important structures are located at or near the orbital rims. The supra-orbital and supra-and infratrochlear nerves emerge in close proximity to the supra-orbital rim, whereas the infra-orbital nerve, which provides sensations to the upper anterior teeth, the lateral nose, and the upper lip, emerges through the infra-orbital foramen, which is just below the infra-orbital rim. The medial canthal ligament, a well-formed structure which maintains the position of the globe medially, is attached to anterior and posterior lacrimal crests by means of its two components. The lateral canthal ligament is a band of fibrous tissue which inserts into the lateral wall of the orbit below and behind the fronto-zygomatic suture. Disruption of the medial canthal ligament results in increased intercanthal distance, and is termed traumatic telecanthus; this would result in a mongoloid slant. Lateral canthal ligamental displacement would give an anti-mongoloid slant.

The lacrimal apparatus, the extra-ocular muscles, the globe, the optic nerve, and the contents (nerves and blood-vessels) of the superior orbital fissure are important anatomical struc-

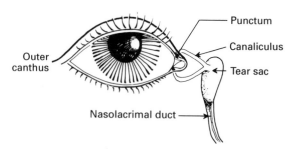

Fig. 7.2 • Anatomy of the lacrimal apparatus.

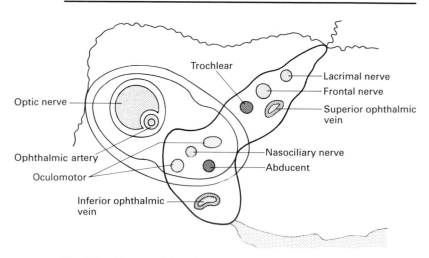

Fig. 7.3 • Nerves of the orbital apex and the superior orbital fissure.

tures which can be involved in malar orbital trauma (Figs 7.2 and 7.3).

Aetiology

The incidence of malar orbital fractures may make up anything from 20 per cent to 60 per cent of all maxillofacial trauma. These fractures can occur alone or in combination with other midface fractures.

The majority of these fractures are caused by interpersonal assault; the next most common cause is sporting accidents, and road-traffic incidents rank only third in prevalence (Table 7.1).

MacLennan in 1977 commented on the aetiology of maxillofacial trauma as 'a rather sober reflection on the increasing violence in the society in which we live today'.

In a recent prospective study Al Quarainy *et al.* (1991*b*) found that 90 per cent of patients with malar orbital fractures sustained ocular injuries of varying severities. Of those 12 per cent experienced very severe eye injuries.

Classification

The main reasons for classifying fractures are to allow description of the injury in a simplified way and to aid in the establishment of a treatment plan. Several classifications are available for malar fractures. These are based on the type of bony displacement. These systems tend to confuse the novice in maxillofacial trauma, and thus to defeat their purpose. The following classification is based on anatomy, and can be easily described over the phone without any confusion (Table 7.2).

Assessment

- **General assessment Ophthalmic assessment Extraoral examination Intraoral examination**

General assessment

The most important initial assessment of the malar orbital fracture is the examination of the eye. Since the majority of these fractures involve associated ocular injury ophthalmic referral should be considered at the earliest opportunity. The Canniesburn occular trauma score recommended by Al

Table 7.1 • Aetiology of malar orbital fractures

Assault	— 55 per cent
Sports	— 20 per cent
Road-traffic accidents	— 15 per cent
Others	— 10 per cent

Table 7.2 • Anatomical classification of malar orbital fractures

1. Fracture with no displacement
2. Fracture displacement of the lateral wall of the antrum
3. Fracture displacement of the infra-orbital rim
4. Fracture displacement of the zygomatic arch
5. Fracture displacement of the lateral orbital rim
6. Fracture displacement of the supra-orbital rim
7. Fracture displacement of the medial rim
8. 'Blow-in' fracture
9. 'Blow-out' fracture
10. Comminuted fracture

Qurainy et al. (1991a) (Table 7.3) is a very helpful screening aid, and similar to the Glasgow Coma Scale for head injury.

The general assessment also includes the history of the injury, past medical history, and present medication. Knowledge of any anticoagulant therapy is important in the management of intra-orbital bleeding.

The specific examination for malar orbital fractures involves detailed inspection and palpation, both extra- and intraorally. Intraoral percussion is sometimes also helpful in the diagnosis.

The patient should be inspected and palpated from both the front and back for any localized clinical features. The clinical manifestations tend to vary according to the time interval which has elapsed since the injury, its severity, and the extent to which the associated structures are involved. The following signs and symptoms are described on the basis of the anatomical structures of the malar orbital region (Figs 7.4, 7.5, and 7.6).

Ophthalmic assessment

Table 7.3 • Ophthalmic referral

Clinical findings as a sequel to injury		Score
Visual acuity	6/6 or better	0
	6/9–6/12	4
	6/18–6/24	8
	6/36 or less	12
	No perception of light	16
Malar fracture	Comminuted	3
	Blow-out	3
	Other	0
Motility disorder		
(e.g. diplopia or post-traumatic squint)		
	Present	3
	Absent	0
Retrograde and post-traumatic amnesia		
	Present	5
	Absent	0

Final score

If the final score is 11, then add 1:
(a) if sex is female.
(b) if age is 30–39.
(c) if cause of injury is a road-traffic accident.

Total score

If total score = 0–4: Do not refer.
= 5–11: Consider routine referral.
= 12+: Consider urgent referral.

Extraoral examination

A: Periorbital structures
- Periorbital oedema
- Circumorbital ecchymosis
- Subconjunctival ecchymosis
- Surgical emphysema

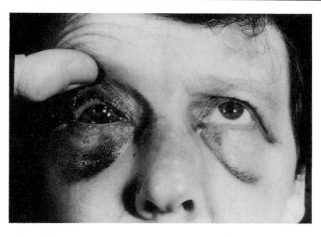

Fig. 7.4 • A 42-year-old female patient sustained fracture of the malar orbital complex, demonstrating right periorbital oedema, bilateral circumorbital ecchymosis, right subconjunctival ecchymosis, narrowing of the right palpebral fissure, drop in pupillary level, and a flat malar prominence.

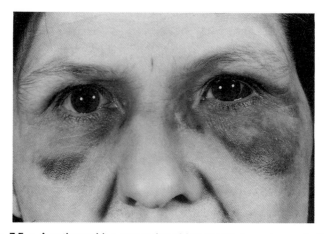

Fig. 7.5 • A patient with a seven-day-old malar fracture, demonstrating resolving swelling and bruising. Note that the subconjunctival ecchymosis will remain red in colour until it disappears.

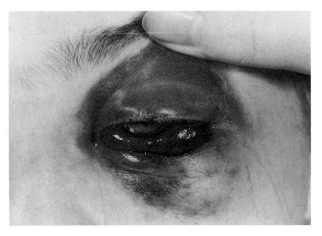

Fig. 7.6 • Close-up view of the left eye, which demonstrates gross ecchymosis.

B: The eyelids
- Abnormality of the palpebral fissure
- Ptosis or pseudoptosis
- Lacerations or abrasions

C: The ligaments
- Traumatic telecanthus
- Mongoloid slant
- Anti-mongoloid slant

D: The globe
- Pupillary level and size
- Enophthalmos
- Traumatic exophthalmos
- Visual acuity
- Motility disorder
- Diplopia
- Direct and consensual reflexes

E: Intra-ocular injuries
- Corneal abrasion
- Hyphaema

- Presence of foreign body
- Iridodialysis
- Choroidal tear
- Retinal detachment
- Commotio retinae

F: The lacrimal apparatus
- Epiphora
- Damage to puncta
- Damage to nasolacrimal duct

G: Nerves
- Anaesthesia or paraesthesia of:
  —supra-orbital nerve
  —supratrochlear nerve
  —infra-orbital nerve
  —zygomatico-facial and temporal nerves
- Traumatic optic neuropathy
- Superior orbital fissure syndrome
- Orbital apex syndrome

H: Bony structure
- Tenderness on palpation and/or step deformity at superior margin
- Fronto-zygomatic suture
- Inferior margin
- Nasofrontal and nasomaxillary sutures
- Malar body
- Zygomatic arch
- Zygomatic buttress
- Lateral antral wall

Sometimes a malar arch fracture may impinge on the coronoid process of the mandible and cause trismus.

Intraoral examination

Intraoral examination should always be performed with a gloved hand. The buccal sulcus and the buttress region should be examined for tenderness and step deformity. Percussion of the teeth sometimes provide a clue for a possible fracture. Altered occlusion of the teeth is an indication of an associated maxillary fracture.

Special investigations

- **Plain radiographs   CT scans and MRI   3D reformation**

Box 7.1 **Special investigations**

- Plain radiographs
- Computerized tomography (CT)
- Magnetic Resonance Imaging (MRI)
- 3-dimensional reformation

Plain radiographs

The majority of fractures can be diagnosed with the help of plain radiographs. The most useful radiographic views for malar orbital fractures are:

- 15° occipitomental (Fig. 7.7);
- 35° occipitomental (Fig. 7.8); and
- submento-vertex with reduced exposure (Fig. 7.9) (to demonstrate the zygomatic arches).

Further information may be obtained from:

- a Zonarc MT projection (for ethmoid and maxillary sinuses) (Fig. 7.10); and
- a tomogram (for blow-out fractures) (Fig. 7.11).

McGregor and Campbell's first three lines can be used as an aid to study occipitomental radiographs systematically. It is emphasized that malar orbital fractures should be diagnosed with positive clinical signs rather than by radiographic findings alone. The distance between the zygomatic arch and

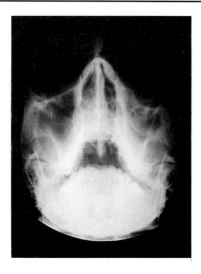

Fig. 7.7 • Radiograph (15° occipitomental view), demonstrating fracture displacement of the infra-orbital rim, malar body, malar arch, and lateral wall.

the top of the coronoid process gives a clue as to the displacement of the malar body.

CT scans and MRI

In the last few years Computerized Tomography (CT) and Magnetic Resonance Imaging (MRI) have been used to a greater extent in the diagnosis of malar orbital fractures. Although magnetic resonance imaging at present is not available in many centres, it has several advantages over CTs; these include excellent soft-tissue contrast, while the bone can also be visualized equally well as dark areas (Figs 7.12 and 7.13). The MR images are not distorted by metallic fixtures. Further, patients with multiple injuries can be placed in the MR chamber without having to tilt the neck, which is necessary in CT in order to obtain direct sections.

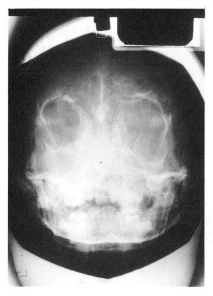

Fig. 7.8 • Radiograph (30° occipitomental view), demonstrating fracture of the left malar bone, with an opaque left antrum.

Reformatted CT scans can be obtained without tilting the patient, but the final scans lack clarity. In years to come MRI will supersede CT as the initial imaging modality in the diagnosis of malar orbital fractures.

3D reformation

Because of improvements in computer sophistication with 3D techniques orbital and globe volumes can be quantified accurately. Mirror images of the unaffected side can be produced for comparison with the affected side. A workstation concept, where the surgeon can interact and quantify the defects, is more useful than obtaining fixed images. However versatile this technique may be, it is less user-friendly in the management of acute maxillofacial trauma, but extremely useful in the correction of the post-traumatic deformity.

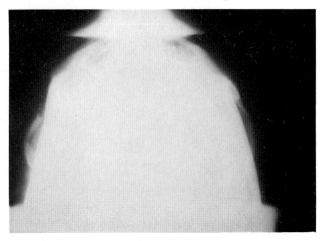

Fig. 7.9 • Submento-vertex radiograph, showing fracture displacement of the malar arch.

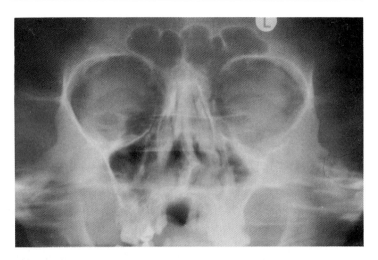

Fig. 7.10 • Zonarc MT projection, showing the sinuses clearly, and also a fracture at the left infra-orbital rim.

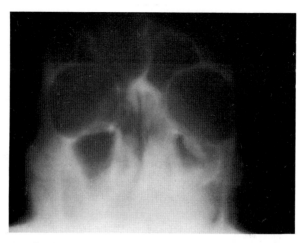

Fig. 7.11 • Orbital tomogram, showing a blow-out fracture of the left orbital floor.

Treatment

- **Initial treatment   Definitive treatment   Postoperative care   Complications**

Initial treatment

When there is a full-thickness laceration of the eyelid or damage to the lacrimal apparatus, definitive treatment should be instituted immediately. For closed malar orbital fractures with swelling and bruising final treatment can be delayed for about 5–7 days. In the mean time, instructions should be given to avoid nose-blowing and smoking. A suitable antibiotic may be prescribed as a prophylaxis.

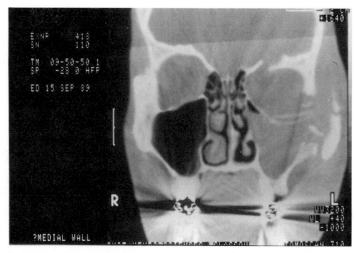

Fig. 7.12 • Coronal CT scan of a comminuted fracture of the left orbit and malar bones. The bone is demonstrated as white areas.

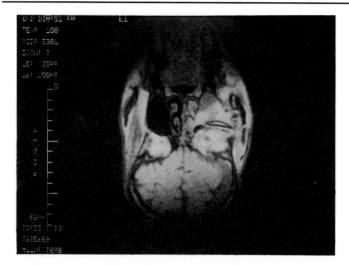

Fig. 7.13 • Coronal MR imaging of the same patient, where the bone is demonstrated as dark areas; the inferior rectus muscle is entrapped into the floor, and also shows fat herniation into the maxillary antrum and ethmoid sinus.

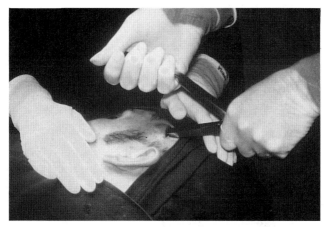

Fig. 7.14 • Gillies temporal incision, with an instrument placed just under the temporalis fascia.

If there is associated ocular trauma or head injury the patient should be admitted and managed accordingly. The Canniesburn ocular trauma scoring system (table 7.3) will be of assistance in deciding whether to refer to an ophthalmologist.

Definitive treatment

Nowadays it is accepted practice that initial treatment is the best opportunity to treat malar orbital fractures. This may involve immediate bone-grafting in order to obtain symmetry and support, in addition to elevation, fixation, and sometimes immobilization. The main rehabilitative process in these injuries is the orthoptic exercises that are undertaken in order to obtain full ocular motility and binocular vision as soon as possible.

Depressed malar fractures can be elevated using a Rowe's malar elevator via a Gillies temporal incision (Fig. 7.14) or

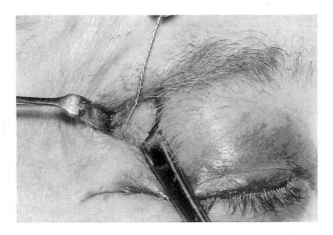

Fig. 7.15 • Wire osteosynthesis at the fronto-zygomatic suture.

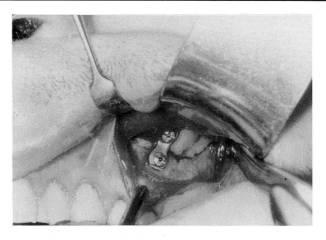

Fig. 7.16 • Intraoral mini-plate osteosynthesis to stabilize a malar fracture.

by inserting a malar hook under the malar body (see Fig. 7.1, p. 136). The Rowe's elevator is inserted under the temporalis fascia to engage the malar arch. Further elevation can be performed through existing lacerations or other surgical incisions. It is a firm belief among many maxillofacial surgeons that early elevation prevents permanent damage to the infraorbital nerve in cases where there is evidence of compression.

If the malar bone is fractured in more than one place a two-point fixation is essential, preferably in a vertical dimension (Figs 7.15, 7.16, 7.17). As in other orthopaedic injuries, either external or internal fixation can be used to immobilize malar fractures. Although the concept of rigid internal fixation is becoming more popular, the surgeon should be aware of other fixation techniques as well (Figs 7.18, 7.19);

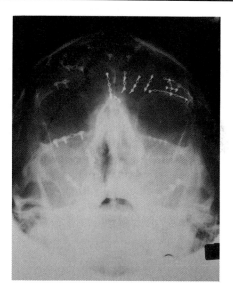

Fig. 7.17 • Occipitomental radiograph, demonstrating micro-plate fixation to the supraorbital rim and orbital roof, and mini-plate fixation to the lateral wall of the orbit.

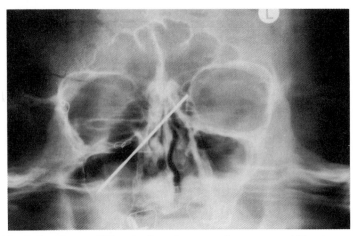

Fig. 7.18 • Zonarc MT projection, demonstrating transnasal Kirschner wire fixation to stabilize a malar fracture.

packing the antrum to support malar orbital fractures is not a very satisfactory technique, as it causes more complications than benefits. The surgical access to the malar orbital region can be obtained via the following approaches:

- a fronto-zygomatic incision;
- a crow-foot incision;
- a blepharoplasty incision;
- an infra-orbital incision;
- a transconjunctival incision;
- a bicoronal flap; and
- an intraoral buttress incision.

The orbital rims and the malar bone fractures are stabilized using the above-mentioned internal or external fixation techniques. If the orbital wall fractures demonstrate soft-tissue herniation or entrapment the contents should be retrieved and the walls should be reconstructed using autogenous (bone, cartilage) or alloplastic (silastic sheets) materials. It is also a useful practice to prescribe a short course of steroid therapy to reduce orbital swelling.

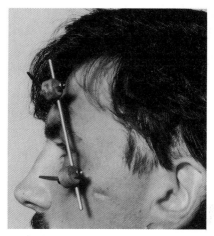

Fig. 7.19 • External pin fixation is used to stabilize a comminuted left malar complex.

Postoperative care

After surgery the following instructions are given to the ward staff:

- nurse upright;
- make regular eye observation; and;
- avoid and discourage nose-blowing.

Complications

The most important perioperative or immediate postoperative complication of malar orbital surgery is the retrobulbar haemorrhage. The clinical features of this problem are retro-orbital pain of increasing severity, proptosis, a tense hard eye with a dilating pupil, ophthalmoplegia, decreasing visual acuity, and a pale optic disc. Treatment is both surgical and medical; both must be commenced simultaneously. Decompression of the globe is the first essential procedure. This can be carried out through existing incisions or through an elective infra-orbital incision. A lateral canthotomy allows the globe to move freely.

Intravenous acetazolamide 500 mg and hydrocortisone 100 mg are the most useful medical measures. A rapid infusion of 20 per cent mannitol 200 ml has also been recommended. When vision improves prednisolone 60 mg a day and acetazolamide 500 mg twice a day should be continued for one week.

Other complications are lower-lid ectropion, persistent diplopia, enophthalmos, and a flat malar prominence.

Further reading

Al-Qurainy, I. A. Titterington, D. M., Dutrton, G. N., Stassen, L. F. A., Moos, K. F., and El-Attar, A. (1991a). Mid facial fractures and the eye: the development of a system for detecting patients at risk. *British Journal of Oral and Maxillofacial Surgery*, **29**, 363–7.

Al-Qurainy, I. A., Stassen, L. F. A., Dutton, G. N., Moos, K. F., and El-Attar, A. (1991b). The characteristics of midfacial fractures and the association with ocular injury: a prospective study. *British Journal of Oral and Maxillofacial Surgery*, **29**, 291–301.

MacLennan W. A. (1977). Fractures of the malar (zygomatic) bone. *Journal of the Royal College* (Edinburgh), **22** (3), 187–96.

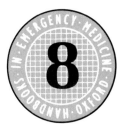

Oral medicine and salivary gland disease

Key points in oral medicine

1 The persistence of any ulcer for over three weeks should raise the question of malignancy and lead to appropriate referral, investigation, and treatment.

ORAL MEDICINE

- Ulceration Stomatitis White
  lesions Malignancy Pigmented lesions HIV infection

Ulceration

- Specific ulceration Gingival ulceration

Acute ulceration of the mouth may be generalized, when it is termed *stomatitis*, or localized and due to specific trauma, or may primarily affect the gingivae, as in acute ulcerative gingivitis.

Specific ulceration

Traumatic ulcers may result from denture flanges, toothbrushing, and burns (Fig. 8.1), and have to be differentiated from ulcers arising from other causes, particularly malignancy. The three stage of syphilis may also cause oral

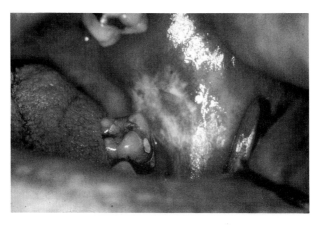

Fig. 8.1 • A chemical burn ulcer—in this case caused by aspirin placed in the buccal sulcus against a painful tooth. (See colour plate section.)

ulceration, but syphilitic ulcers are now much less commonly seen than in the past. Squamous cell carcinoma is responsible for the majority of cases of intraoral malignancy, and its most frequent presentation is that of a solitary ulcerative lesion.

Gingival ulceration

Acute necrotizing ulcerative gingivitis is a rapidly progressive infection destroying the periodontal tissues, typically starting at the tips of the interdental papillae, and is associated with pain, gingival bleeding, and an unpleasant smell. The latter is due to the anaerobic infection causing the disease, and the response to metronidazole 400 mg three times a day for five days is excellent, but needs to be followed by dental scaling and improvement in oral hygiene.

Stomatitis

• **Infective stomatitis   Non-infective stomatitis**

This may be infective or non-infective.

Infective stomatitis

Viral stomatitis

Viral stomatitis is predominantly caused by *Herpes simplex*, although Coxsackie A (hand, foot, and mouth) may also present as a generalized stomatitis. Primary herpetic stomatitis causes a widespread vesicular eruption, especially on the hard palate and the dorsum of the tongue, which quickly ruptures to form small painful ulcers. It is seen in all ages, but particularly in children, and often in association with red and swollen gums, systemic upset, and cervical lymphadenopathy. The lesions are contagious, but usually clear up in 7 to 10 days, and treatment is to prevent dehydration in the young, with provision of pain relief, and in severe cases the prescription of acyclovir (Fig. 8.2).

   Herpes zoster causes shingles, and may affect the trigeminal nerve, producing the characteristic rash and pain in the distribution of one or more of its divisions. This infec-

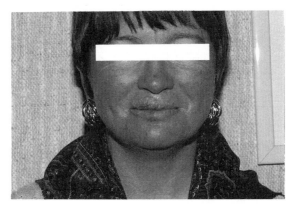

Fig. 8.2 • Lip lesions of *Herpes simplex*. (See colour plate section.)

tion may be difficult to differentiate from severe toothache before the rash has erupted, and again acyclovir is the appropriate treatment.

Fungal stomatitis

Candida albicans may present in several clinical guises intraorally.

Thrush is the commonest presentation, with creamy white patches on the oral mucosa which rub off easily to leave an erythematous or raw surface. Topical antifungal therapy is effective, and simple haematological investigations may be indicated, as this condition is frequently seen in patients with other diseases or who are immunocompromised.

Candidal infection may be confined to the denture-bearing area of the mouth, and there cause a generalized erythema, with or without plaques of thrush, when it is known as 'denture stomatitis'. Topical antifungal treatment to the soft tissues and thorough cleansing (hypochlorite 1 per cent) of the dentures is indicated.

Angular cheilitis or stomatitis is common to many oral candidal infections, and varies in severity from reddening of the corners of the mouth to frank ulceration (Fig. 8.3).

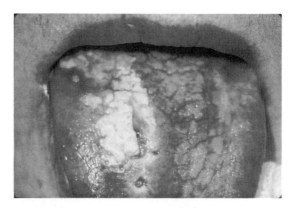

Fig. 8.3 • Chronic candidiasis of the right side of the tongue. (See colour plate section.)

The other important presentation of *Candida albicans* in the mouth is that of chronic hyperplastic candidosis, whose plaques cannot be easily rubbed off; and often a biopsy is required for differential diagnosis of this type of leukoplakia.

Non-infective stomatitis

Recurrent aphthae. The commonest form of recurrent ulceration in the mouth is minor aphthae, but the herpetiform and major types may also be seen.

The salient feature is the history, which is often of several years' duration; and ulceration occurs on a regular basis, with multiple small ulcers erupting on the buccal mucosa, the lips, the sulci, and the lateral border of the tongue (Fig. 8.4).

Some of these patients have underlying haematological deficiency states, for instance vitamin B_{12}, folate, and iron, and this issue may be investigated alongside active management of the ulcers. Treatment of the condition is preventive, using steroids topically (corlan pellets or adcortyl paste) before the eruption of the ulcers, or therapeutic when the ulcers have erupted, using chlorhexidine or tetracycline mouth washes. Behçet's syndrome produces oral lesions closely resembling aphthae, but these are symptoms of a

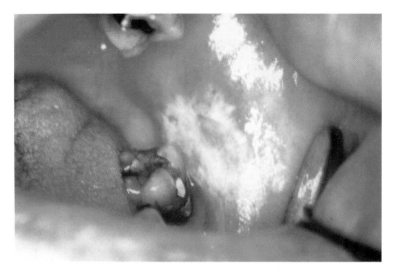

Plate 8.1 A chemical burn ulcer—in this case caused by aspirin placed in the buccal sulcus against a painful tooth.

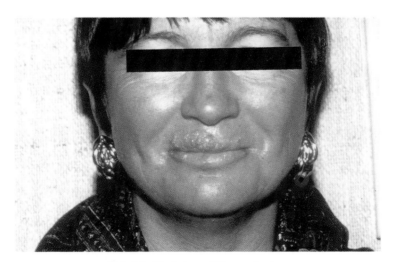

Plate 8.2 Lip lesions of *Herpes simplex*.

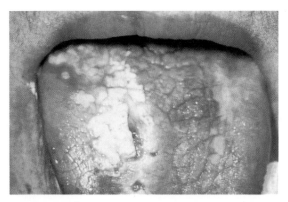

Plate 8.3   Chronic candidiasis of the right side of the tongue.

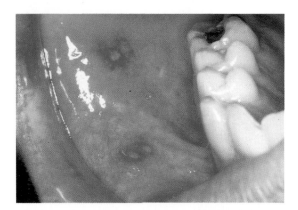

Plate 8.4   Minor aphthæ seen in recurrent oral ulceration.

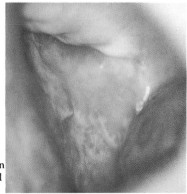

Plate 8.5   White striae of lichen planus on the buccal mucosa.

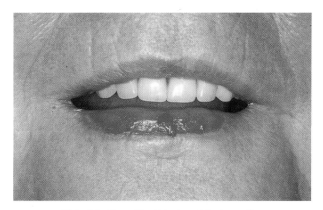

Plate 8.6 Pemphigoid lesion of the lower lip.

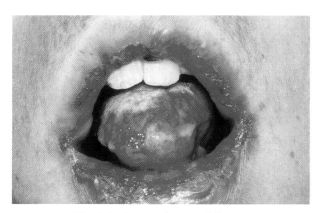

Plate 8.7 Acute erythema multiforme.

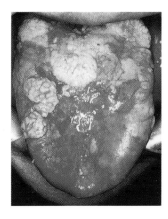

Plate 8.8 Gross leukoplakia of the tongue.

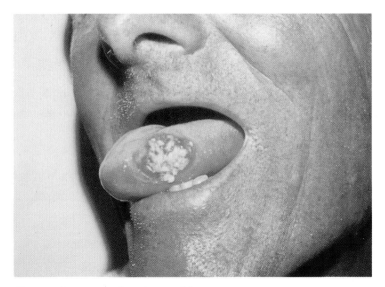

Plate 8.9   Squamous cell carcinoma of the tongue.

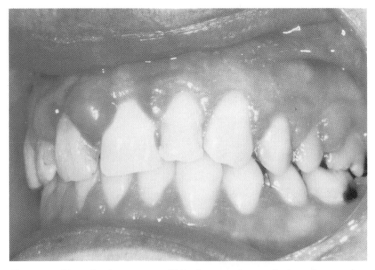

Plate 8.10   Gingival enlargement and bleeding seen in acute leukaemia.

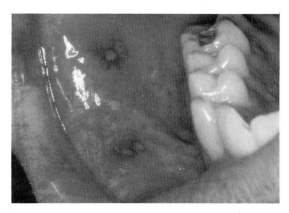

Fig. 8.4 • Minor aphthae seen in recurrent oral ulceration. (See colour plate section.)

multisystem disorder affecting the eyes, joints, and skin.

Other systemic diseases may present in the mouth, either alone or in conjunction with a skin eruption. Examples include lichen planus, with its white striae, erosions, and atrophic areas, particularly on the buccal mucosa; pemphigus vulgaris; and mucous membrane pemphigoid, which presents as intraoral bullae whose fragility is such that they

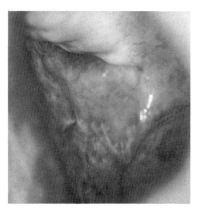

Fig. 8.5 • White striae of lichen planus on the buccal mucosa. (See colour plate section.)

often break down and present as diffuse erosions (Figs 8.5 and 8.6).

Acute erythema multiforme may also present on the skin, but the mouth is predominantly affected. Said to be precipitated by certain infections (herpes and mycoplasma) and drugs (barbiturates and sulphonamides), most cases how-

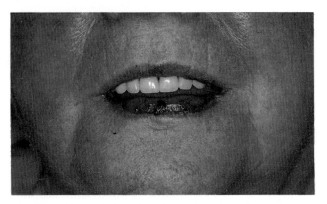

Fig. 8.6 • Pemphigoid lesion of the lower lip. (See colour plate section.)

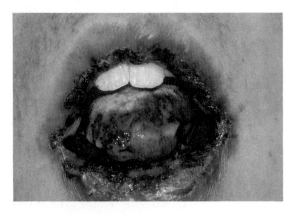

Fig. 8.7 • Acute erythema multiforme. (See colour plate section.)

ever fail to provide a positive history. Fever and systemic upset precede the oral eruption of erosions and erythema, strikingly seen as swollen, ulcerated, bleeding, and crusting lips. Skin and conjunctival lesions may occur, and treatment is supportive and directed to the prevention of complications such as infection and ocular damage (Fig. 8.7).

White lesions

The term *leukoplakia* is given to any white lesion for which a diagnosis cannot be made, and does not imply any histological connotation.

Conditions previously mentioned which present as white patches include lichen planus, candidosis, and such traumatic lesions as cheek-biting and chemical burns. The term 'leukoplakia' has become associated with malignancy or premalignancy, and although it is true that any white lesion should be viewed with suspicion until diagnosis, the majority will have no malignant potential.

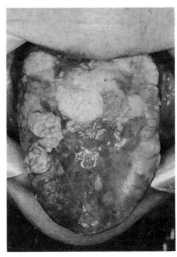

Fig. 8.8 • Gross leukoplakia of the tongue. (See colour plate section.)

The clinical presentation of leukoplakia is varied, and there is no direct correlation of appearance to malignancy; however, assessment of aetiological factors such as smoking and alcohol, clinical examination, and biopsy are necessary steps in the management of these lesions (Fig. 8.8).

Erythematous and speckled areas associated with leukoplakia are viewed with greater suspicion.

Malignancy

The incidence of oral squamous cell carcinoma appears to be rising, particularly in the 35–55-year age-group, and carries an overall 5-year survival of less than 50 per cent. Early diagnosis is of great importance, and any ulcer or lesion which persists for more than a few weeks should be expertly examined and investigated appropriately.

Squamous cell carcinoma of the oral cavity generally present as chronic indurated ulcers with typical raised edges and central granulation, but can occasionally present as red or white lumps or fissures.

Treatment is primarily by surgery or radiotherapy, or a combination of both (Fig. 8.9).

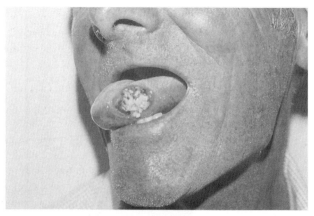

Fig. 8.9 • Squamous cell carcinoma of the tongue. (See colour plate section.)

Box 8.1 **Squamous cell carcinoma: aetiology and presentation**

Aetiology	**Presentation**
Tobacco/alcohol	Persistent ulcer with raised
Premalignant lesions:	everted edges, induration,
dysplastic mucosa	and central granulation.
leukoplakia	Occasionally palatal or
lichen planus	alveolar lumps and tongue
submucous fibrosis	fissures.
tertiary syphilis	

Pigmented lesions

Mucosal pigmentation due to racial origin is to be expected, but may also occur in a small percentage of Caucasians, and can involve both oral mucosa and gingivae. Endocrine disturbances such as Addison's disease or oral contraceptives may increase melanin production, and haemorrhagic disorders, for example purpura, may produce small petechiae or widespread ecchymosis, which unlike haemangiomas will not blanch on pressure.

Malignant melanoma is rare in the mouth. Other uncommon causes of oral pigmentation include Peutz–Jeghers syndrome and tattooing.

HIV infection

The oral cavity is a frequent site of clinical signs and symptoms of patients with HIV infection. Like TB of old, HIV may mimic a wide variety of pathological conditions, but the most common oral presentations seen are ulceration, candidosis, hairy leukoplakia, acute necrotizing ulcerative gingivitis and other periodontal disorders, and Kaposi's sarcoma.

Immunosupression of any cause will also allow a variety of infections, for example viral, to present, and the haematological disturbances of the acute leukaemias may be seen first in the mouth, with gingival enlargement and bleeding (Fig. 8.10).

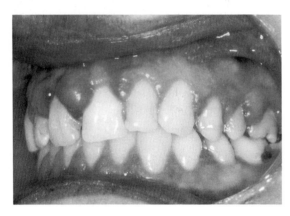

Fig. 8.10 • Gingival enlargement and bleeding seen in acute leukaemia. (See colour plate section.)

SALIVARY GLAND DISEASE

• **Infection   Obstruction   Neoplasia**

Individual glands are commonly affected, but disease may also be generalized and affect all salivary tissue in and around the mouth.

Infection

Viral infection

Viral salivary gland infection is classically illustrated by the condition of mumps, due to paramyovirus, which affects the parotid or occasionally the submandibular glands bilaterally following a three-week inoculation period. It is usually painful, with associated inflammation of the ducts; but the

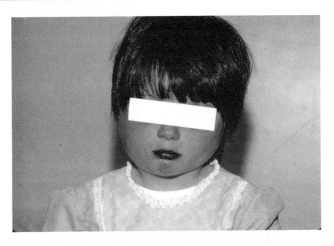

Fig. 8.11 • Bilateral parotid enlargement in mumps.

treatment is symptomatic. Viral infections may rarely also be unilateral and caused by other viruses, such as echo, coxsackie, or EBV (Fig. 8.11).

Bacterial infection

Bacterial salivary gland infection is usually due to the ascent of microorganisms up the duct of the gland, or rarely to haematogenous spread (TB). This is usually associated with dehydration and non-functioning of the gland. Its presentation is that of an inflamed painful swelling of an individual gland, with a purulent discharge from its duct, which can be cultured; but the usual infecting organisms, viz. staphylococci, streptococci, and various anaerobes, can be targeted with appropriate antibiotics from the outset.

Surgical drainage is reserved for those cases which fail to respond to antibiotics, mouthwashes, and the encouragement of drainage via the duct.

Following treatment it is important to investigate the gland for local and correctable abnormalities which may predispose to recurrence of the problem, for example duct strictures.

Obstruction

As in any duct and gland, obstruction may be extrinsic, for example, through neoplasia; within the walls of the duct, for example, by stricture; or within the duct, for example, through the presence of calculi or mucous plugs (Fig. 8.12).

Calculi are the main cause of glandular obstruction, and are seen most frequently in the submandibular glands. Swelling of the gland occurs at times of salivary stimulation, particularly mealtimes, and may be painful; but the obstruction is usually transient. Recurrent episodes of obstruction will lead to damage to the gland, which can become irreversible.

Plain radiography will detect 60–80 per cent of calculi, but sialography is required for radiolucent stones or strictures.

Surgical removal of the obstruction is usually necessary, either from the duct, if the stone is at the orifice or anteriorly placed, so leaving the gland intact; or by removal of the affected gland, if the obstruction is intraglandular or the gland is badly scarred by repeated episodes of obstruction or inflammation.

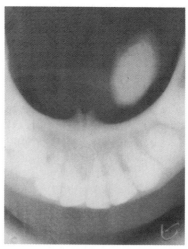

Fig. 8.12 • Radiograph of a submandibular duct stone.

Obstruction or damage to minor salivary glands or their ducts may produce mucoceles or mucus-extravasation cysts, seen most commonly on the lower lip as a dome-shaped bluish swelling. Treat by surgical excision or cryotherapy.

Neoplasia

There are a wide range of neoplastic salivary gland swellings, and the majority are benign. Some 75 per cent of swellings are pleomorphic salivary adenomas, particularly in the parotid and the palate. Normally these swellings have a long clinical history (years) and cause few or no symptoms, so the presence of a short history, pain, lymphadenopathy, or nerve (VII) involvement should alert the clinician to the possibility of malignancy. Salivary swellings in the sublingual and submandibular glands should particularly be viewed with suspicion.

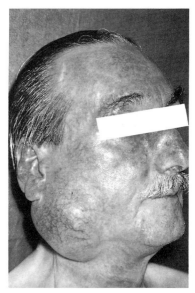

Fig. 8.13 • Salivary neoplasia of the right parotid gland.

After investigations for example (CT, MRI, ultrasound, and fine-needle aspiration) surgical excision of the mass is usually indicated, and may be local, as in the palate or lip, or may involve the removal of the bulk or the whole of the gland, as in superficial parotidectomy (Fig. 8.13).

Index